MORTALITY DECLINE AND ITS DEMOGRAPHIC EFFECTS IN LATIN AMERICA

Mortality Decline and Its Demographic Effects In Latin America

EDUARDO E. ARRIAGA

Institute of International Studies
University of California, Berkeley

Standard Book Number 87725-306-4
Library of Congress Card Number 79-630857

FOREWORD

In another book in this series--New Life Tables for Latin American Populations in the Nineteenth and Twentieth Centuries--Dr. Arriaga provided basic data for a more accurate history of mortality in Latin America. Now he has used that material to delineate the history itself and to analyze its demographic effects. Among other things, he has shown that the drop in death rates has been even more rapid than was previously thought, thus strengthening the view that it was the fastest drop ever experienced by a major world region. As for the demographic consequences, he shows that these are equally arresting.

What happens with a fall in mortality depends not only on how far but also on how fast it falls. In the case of Latin America, the fall has been so rapid, compared to an equal decline in the past history of more advanced regions, that other aspects of demographic behavior have had little time to respond. Fertility has remained far higher, at given levels of mortality, than it did in Europe or the United States. This fact has caused the rate of natural increase to exceed anything ever known before in a major region. Yet this is not the whole story. In Latin America the rapid decline in mortality has tended to increase fertility, in the sense of the number of offspring per woman. This effect is usually overlooked, because the quick mortality decline has also, along with enhanced fertility, enlarged the proportion of children in the population and thus reduced the crude birth rate. As a consequence, the present rate of natural increase, high as it is, understates the demographic prospect. The young age structure hangs like a cloud over the future.

Owing to the high ratio of children already in the population, a reduction in age-specific fertility rates would fail for decades to produce a commensurate reduction in the crude birth rate. For the same reason, further reduction in age-specific death rates will produce disproportionately low crude rates--rates far lower than in industrialized societies at the same level of mortality. The result is that in Latin America the reduction in marital fertility envisioned by family planners, even if accomplished, will not have much effect on the present rate of population growth.

This and other sobering findings emerge from Dr. Arriaga's imaginative and ingenious analysis of demographic interrelationships. Those who have generously supported the research that has gone into the study--to whom the author makes specific acknowledgment--are to be congratulated as well as thanked for their encouragement of highly relevant basic science. This is the fourth volume to come from IPUR's program of studies in comparative Latin American demography. Others will follow.

Kingsley Davis

International Population and Urban Research
University of California, Berkeley
February 17, 1970

ACKNOWLEDGMENTS

This monograph is based on my Ph.D. dissertation and so I wish to thank the members of the committee, Professors Kingsley Davis (Department of Sociology), Nathan Keyfitz (Department of Demography) and Chin Long Chiang (School of Public Health), for the time they dedicated to advising me. Especially I am grateful to Dr. Kingsley Davis, chairman of the committee and Chairman of International Population and Urban Research, for his invaluable suggestions throughout all chapters and earlier drafts of the study.

I wish also to thank Judith Clark, who is also at IPUR, for her efforts in editing and typing my drafts and for helping with the manuscript in its final dissertation form. In addition, I wish to thank Neda Tomasevich of the Department of Demography, who did the first editing of the present version of the monograph; Paul Gilchrist, of the Institute of International Studies, who edited the monograph in its final form; and Bojana Ristich, who typed the final monograph.

The work was generously supported by research and training grants. A part of the support came from two research funds given to IPUR, one directly by the Rockefeller Foundation and the other by the Institute of International Studies at the University of California from its own Ford Foundation grant. Both of these gifts to IPUR were for comparative research in Latin American demography. Another part of the support was received from two training grants to the Department of Demography, one from the Ford Foundation and the other from the National Institute of General Medical Sciences (5 T01 GM01240). Without these financial aids, the research underlying the monograph could not have been accomplished.

Finally, I am grateful to my wife, Regina, for her help and encouragement.

To all these, many thanks.

Eduardo E. Arriaga

International Population and Urban Research
University of California
February 1970

CONTENTS

LIST OF TABLES

LIST OF FIGURES

PART I

PURPOSES OF THE STUDY AND SOURCES OF DATA

Chapter I

INTRODUCTION

The present study focuses on population change in Latin America during the past one hundred years, with primary emphasis on the period from 1930 to 1960. This latter period has been chosen for detailed analysis because of its central importance for understanding the demographic evolution of current Latin American populations. It was during this period that profound changes in mortality produced the conditions which have led to the serious demographic problems Latin America faces today.

Knowledge regarding the population of Latin America prior to the nineteenth century remains somewhat vague and unreliable. Before the 1800's, censuses were taken infrequently, permitting only regional estimates and rather gross speculations as to the total population of the area.[1] More precise census enumerations were initiated during the nineteenth century within the most populated countries, and estimates of the total population of the Latin American area since then have become increasingly accurate. The total population of Latin America around 1800 is estimated to have been between 15 and 35 million, and in 1850, between 30 and 50 million.[2]

The population of the region in 1900 is estimated to have been 65 million.[3] Since then, its growth has been rapid and has tended to accelerate, as can be seen from the table below.

---

[1]Angel Rosenblat, La Poblacion Indigena y el Mestizaje en America (Buenos Aires: Editorial Nova, Biblioteca Americanista, 1954); Walter Wilcox, "Increase in the Population of the Earth and of the Continents," International Migrations (Washington, D.C.: National Bureau of Economic Research, 1931), 2: 33-82.

[2]John D. Durand, "World Population Estimates, 1750-2000," World Population Conference, 1965, 4 vols. (New York: United Nations, 1967), 2: 17-22.

[3]Ibid.

INTRODUCTION

Table I

LATIN AMERICAN POPULATION

Year	Population (millions)	Average Annual Geometric Growth Rate (thousands)
1900	65	
		17
1930	108	
		19
1940	130	
		23
1950	163	
		27
1960	213	

Source: United Nations, Demographic Yearbook 1967 (New York, 1968), p. 97.

International migration to Latin America was the cause of significant population growth in the nineteenth century, but since 1930 it has been negligible.[4] Mortality and fertility have become, without doubt, the major determinants of the rapid population growth during recent decades. The difference between birth and death rates resulted in a growth rate of 32 per thousand in 1960.

Since in the past fertility remained practically constant at a very high level, the rapid mortality decline must be pointed to as the cause of the extremely high natural growth rates registered for Latin American populations in recent years. The rapidly reduced mortality together with continued high birth rates have produced an overall rate of natural population growth heretofore unparalleled in human history.[5]

---

[4] Karl Gotz, Auswandern? (Friedrich Vorwerk Verlag Stuttgart, 1951); United Nations, Sex and Age of International Migrants: Statistics for 1918-1947 (New York, 1953) and Demographic Yearbook 1959.

[5] Carmen Miro, "The Population of Latin America," Demography, I, No. 1 (1964): 15-41; United Nations, Human Resources of Central America, Panama, and Mexico, 1950-1980, prepared by Luis J. Ducoff (ST/TAD/K/LAT/1, E/CN.12/548) [New York, 1960] and The Population of South America, 1950-1980 (ST/SDA/Series A, Population Studies No. 21) [New York, 1955]; Kingsley Davis, "Population and Resources

Historically, the vast majority of the world's population has lived in a state of extreme poverty, at least in terms of our contemporary conception of this condition. In general, the poorest populations grew relatively slowly, while the populations in economically more advanced countries expanded more rapidly. But none had natural growth rates exceeding 15 per thousand.[6] Today, by contrast, populations in the poorest nations are growing considerably faster than those in any other countries in history. Thus, whereas previously the richest countries were populating the world fastest, at present the poorest countries have the highest rates of population growth.[7] The nations of Latin America belong to this latter group. A very high proportion of Latin Americans live in very poor social and economic conditions; at the same time, their numbers are growing at an extremely fast pace.

Modern developed countries have reduced both mortality and fertility in the process of industrialization. The reduction of mortality has been attributed to improved nutrition[8] and innovations in medical care, which are consequences of technological and economic development.[9] The reduction in fertility has been

---

in the Americas," Proceedings of the Inter-American Conference on Conservation of Renewable Natural Resources (Denver: September 7-20, 1948), pp. 88-96, and "Population Trends and Policies in Latin America," in Some Economic Aspects of Post War Inter-American Relations (Austin: Institute of Latin American Studies, University of Texas, 1946).

[6] Perhaps the only exception was the United States before 1900, when quite high birth rates were registered. Since 1900 the U.S. has had natural growth rates lower than 15 per thousand, although the total population has grown faster due to international migration (see U.S. Department of Commerce, Bureau of the Census, Historical Statistics of the United States, Colonial Times to 1957 [Washington, D.C., 1961]). The population of Australia has also grown faster than 15 per thousand per year, but because of international migration.

[7] See Kingsley Davis, "The Unpredicted Pattern of Population Change," Annals of the American Academy of Political and Social Science, 305 (May 1956): 53-59.

[8] Thomas McKeown and R.G. Record, "Reasons for the Declining of Mortality in England and Wales during the Nineteenth Century," Population Studies, 16 (Nov. 1962): 94-122.

[9] Warren S. Thompson, Population Problems, 4th ed. (New York: McGraw-Hill Book Co., 1953), pp. 73-85.

attributed to the change in reproductive motivation resulting from altered social roles.[10]

The situation in the presently developing countries, such as those of Latin America, is quite different. Mortality decline and economic and technological development do not appear to be closely related; it is obvious, at least, that mortality rates of these countries have declined much more rapidly than their economies have developed.[11] At the same time, measures to reduce fertility seem to have been almost totally absent.

If a population parameter undergoes great changes (as great as the mortality reduction in the case of Latin America), interactions among the other population parameters inevitably result. In most cases, the parameter changes will not cancel out, but rather will produce demographic changes affecting the whole society. For instance, the decline of mortality directly affects the age structure of a population, which in turn influences not only the potential labor force, but also educational needs. Mortality decline also directly affects the duration of marital unions, which are closely related to fertility. An increase in surviving children following upon a decline of mortality will produce rural-urban migration if cultivatable land is limited. It is necessary, therefore, in the present case to analyze the trends of demographic variables and their impact on social and economic conditions to fully understand contemporary Latin American populations.

This study is an attempt to discover the reasons behind an unprecedented mortality decline unaccompanied by substantial economic development. The following questions will be posed: What were the principal features of the mortality decline and its consequences? Why did fertility apparently not react to the

---

[10] Kingsley Davis: Human Society, 19th ed. (New York: The Macmillan Co., 1965), pp. 551-617; "The Sociology of Demographic Behavior," in Robert Merton, Leonard Broom, and Leonard Cottrell, eds., Sociology Today, Problems and Prospects (New York: Basic Books, Inc., 1959), pp. 309-333; "The Theory of Change and Response in Modern Demographic History," Population Index, 29, No. 4 (Oct. 1963): 345-366; and (with Judith Blake) "Social Structure and Fertility: An Analytic Framework," Economic Development and Cultural Change, 4 (April 1956): 211-235.

[11] George Stolnitz, "Recent Mortality Trends in Latin America, Asia and Africa," Population Studies, XIX, No. 2 (Nov. 1965): 117-138; Eduardo Arriaga and Kingsley Davis, "The Pattern of Mortality Change in Latin America," Demography, 6, No. 3 (August 1969): 223-242.

mortality decline? What social and economic changes resulted from this particular relationship between mortality and fertility?[12] The study will then analyze how these populations would have developed had they followed European population trends.

To accomplish this kind of analysis is not an easy task. The historical study of mortality in Latin America is hampered by the scarcity and inaccuracy of available information. It is thus understandable why few preceding studies have dealt with the problem of mortality change.[13] Some of the pioneering studies in this area have shown that although mortality rates still appeared to be relatively high, they were declining at a very rapid rate in the whole Latin American continent.[14] Similarly, studies of fertility trends have also been plagued by scanty and unreliable data. It is only recently that historical estimates of crude birth rates have been published for Latin American countries,[15] and that fertility trends during recent decades have been considered.[16]

---

[12]"The consequences of rapidly declining mortality in underdeveloped regions can be understood only in conjunction with what is happening to fertility" (Kingsley Davis, "The Amazing Decline of Mortality in Underdeveloped Areas," American Economic Review 46 [1956]: 314).

[13]Giorgio Mortara, "Estudos sobre a Utilizacao das Estadisticas do Movimiento da Populacao do Brazil," Revista Brasilera de Estadistica, Year II, No. 7 (July-September 1941), pp. 493-538; O. Cabello, J. Vildosola, and M. Latorre, "Tablas de vida para Chile 1920, 1930 y 1940," Revista Chilena de Higiene y Medicina Preventiva VIII, No. 3 (Sept. 1946) and IX, No. 2 (June 1947); B. Becherelle and Jimenez Reyes, "Tablas de vida para Mexico 1893 a 1956," Revista del Instituto de Salubridad y Enfermedades Tropicales XVIII, No. 2 (June 1958): 81-136.

[14]Davis, "Amazing Decline of Mortality"; George Stolnitz, "A Century of International Mortality Trends: I," Population Studies, 9 (July 1955): 24-55.

[15]O. Andrew Collver, Birth Rates in Latin America (Berkeley: Institute of International Studies, University of California, 1965) [Research Series No. 7]; J.R. Rele, Fertility Analysis through Extension of Stable Population Concepts (Berkeley: Institute of International Studies, University of California, 1967) [Population Monograph Series No. 2].

[16]Eduardo Arriaga, "The Effect of the Decline in Mortality on the Gross Reproduction Rate," Milbank Memorial Fund Quarterly, XLV, No. 3 (July 1967): 333-352; Andrew Collver, "Current Trends

INTRODUCTION

The study is divided into five parts. Part I presents the basic data. The principal source is a set of recently published life tables for Latin American countries, which provide the most complete material of this nature currently available.[17] Information on fertility is obtained from estimates of birth rates and official data for recent years.[18]

In Part II the trend of the mortality decline is analyzed. Chapter III charts the general historical mortality trend for Latin America and compares it with the trend registered for European countries. The chapter concludes with an explanation of the differentials in mortality trends of the two areas. In Chapter IV the analysis of Latin American mortality trends is restricted to countries with detailed mortality information since 1930. The most rapid decline in mortality was recorded from this time on in these countries; indices are included which detect age-specific changes for each sex.

In Part III, Chapters V and VI, a final consideration of mortality trends focuses on the estimated effects of the rapid decline in mortality since the 1930's on the age structure of eleven selected Latin American countries. Once these effects are estimated by using a special methodology, an attempt is then made to determine whether or not these changes in age structure have been favorable to economic development and how they have influenced the costs of education.

The following three chapters of Part IV concentrate on the relationship between mortality change and fertility. Chapter VII begins with an analysis of how the decline in mortality has affected the trend in fertility in the eleven selected populations. Then Chile, the only country among those studied to register a decreasing crude birth rate, is analyzed separately. Chapter VIII compares the relationship between mortality and fertility in Latin America with that in Europe. In addition, a set of hypothetical Latin American populations are calculated, based on the assumption that Latin American countries had the same crude birth rates as European countries had in the past at the mortality

---

and Differentials in Fertility as Revealed by Official Data," Milbank Memorial Fund Quarterly, XLVI (July 1968): 30-48.

[17]Eduardo Arriaga, New Life Tables for Latin American Populations in the Nineteenth and Twentieth Centuries (Berkeley: Institute of International Studies, University of California, 1968) [Population Monograph Series No. 3].

[18]The estimates are from Collver, Birth Rates.

levels of Latin American countries. A comparison between the actual and hypothetical populations demonstrates how much better off the Latin American countries would have been today if they had had the mortality-fertility relationship found in Europe. In Chapter IX the hypothetical mortality-fertility trends are studied further to determine whether or not these trends could reasonably have been expected in Latin America.

Part V summarizes some of the principal problems stemming from the rapid mortality decline.

Chapter II

LATIN AMERICAN DATA USED IN THE DEMOGRAPHIC ANALYSIS

An analysis of the effect of mortality change on other demographic parameters requires accurate knowledge of that change. The mortality information should allow not only a determination of historical trends in the general mortality level of a population, but also, at the very least, an analysis of sex and age changes. The present chapter is a discussion of the mortality information used in this study.

A New Set of Life Tables for Latin American Countries

Since a new and more complete set of life tables for Latin America is now available,[1] the study of mortality in Latin America can be expanded both in terms of the historical period covered and the number of countries included. For instance, in the new set of life tables, information for 1900 or earlier has been increased from three life tables for two countries (Brazil 1872-90 and Mexico 1895 and 1900)[2] to twelve life tables for six countries (Bolivia 1900; Brazil 1872, 1890, and 1900; Costa Rica 1864, 1883, and 1892; Guatemala 1893; Mexico 1895 and 1900; and Paraguay 1886 and 1899). Up to 1930 we now have tables for 30 dates, whereas previously there were tables for only 12 dates.[3]

In addition to supplying more historical information, the new life tables appear to be more accurate than the previous ones, especially for the earliest dates, when vital statistics and population information were not very reliable. Most of the earlier life tables were calculated by using classic methods of life table construction, which required death registration and population censuses. An exception is Brazil 1872-90, for which survivor ratios (calculated by using the information of the 1872

---

[1]Arriaga, New Life Tables.

[2]Mortara, "Movimiento da Populacao do Brazil"; Becherelle and Reyes, "Tablas de vida para Mexico."

[3]Arriaga and Davis, "Pattern of Mortality Change."

and 1900 censuses) were used.[4] Although such standard methods of constructing life tables were suitable, the errors which the basic data probably had were inevitably reflected in the results, especially when such data were not evaluated and corrected.[5] Most of the basic data on which conclusions in this study are based is drawn from the newly formulated life tables. Let us consider briefly how the tables were constructed.

Two methods were used. One utilized death and population information and was applied to those dates with accurate information or when the available data allowed an evaluation of the completeness of the censuses and the registers, and thus their correction.[6] This method was applied to Mexico since 1921 and

---

[4]Mortara, "Movimiento da Populacao do Brazil."

[5]United Nations, Demographic Yearbook 1950 (New York, 1951), Table 16, classifies information on death by age groups. Of a total of fifteen Latin American countries, nine warn about the incompleteness of the registers. See also Jorge Somoza, "Trends of Mortality and Expectation of Life in Latin America," Milbank Memorial Fund Quarterly, XLIII, No. 4 (Oct. 1965): 219-233. The author credits only six countries out of twenty with complete registers in the 1960's. For an example of the magnitude of register omission, see Eduardo Arriaga, "New Abridged Life Tables for Peru: 1940, 1950-51 and 1961," Demography, III, No. 1 (July 1966): 218-237.

Several factors have affected the registration of deaths. One is the late date of enforcing registration of deaths by law (United Nations, Handbook of Vital Statistics Methods, Series F, No. 7 [New York, 1955], pp. 20-21). Another is the fee required for the registration of deaths in some countries, such as Venezuela, Haiti, and Bolivia (ibid., pp. 81-82). The organization of the registering system could make it difficult to report deaths (see Eduardo Arriaga, "Rural-Urban Mortality in Developing Countries: An Index for Detecting Rural Underregistration," Demography, IV, No. 1 (December 1967): 90-107).

Because of the scarcity and inaccuracy of data, studies of Latin American mortality have been limited not only in the historical period considered, but also in the number of countries analyzed. See, for instance, Stolnitz, "International Mortality Trends: I," and "Recent Mortality Trends" and Gwendolyn Johnson, "Health Conditions in Rural and Urban Areas of Developing Countries," Population Studies, XVII, No. 3 (March 1964): 292-309.

[6]J. Barral Souto and J. Somoza, "Construcción de una Tabla Abreviada de Mortalidad para la Argentina," Segundo Coloquio de Estadistica (Cordoba, Argentina, 1953).

to Chile, Costa Rica, and Venezuela in the 1960's, because these four were the only countries in the 1960's with sufficient information to permit an evaluation of the statistics. The rest of the life tables--for any date in any country--were constructed by using a new method, based on the Stable Population Theory, which avoids the irregularities of enumeration or misreporting and makes it possible to construct tables even for dates when there was no death registration. The method can be successfully applied to populations considered quasi-stable--that is, populations in which fertility has been practically constant in the past and in which international migration has been negligible. These characteristics are typical of most Latin American populations.

The second method consists of estimating the male and female proportional age distribution in the stable population of the country at the census date. For this determination an estimate of the intrinsic growth rate (the natural growth rate is accepted as a good estimate because of the population characteristics)[7] and a set of model life tables are needed, in addition to the proportional age group distribution between ages 10 and 59.[8] The advantages of using the proportional age distribution between ages 10 and 59 of the actual population as basic data are that (a) the common under- or overenumeration of all ages vanishes, and (b) the usual underenumeration in ages under 10 and overenumeration in ages 60 and over does not affect the result of the life table.[9] These advantages increase the possibility of using censuses where incompleteness would have created problems were another method employed.

The estimation of the proportional age group distribution of the stable population for each country--at each date when a

---

[7]The populations can be considered quasi-stable because of the almost constant fertility and declining mortality rates in the past.

[8]This method was tested in Latin American countries, as well as in Sweden for 1750, 1790, and 1830. The comprehensive information for Chile in 1960 allowed us to construct a life table by using vital statistics and population information. In addition, a life table was constructed by using the method based on stable population. The two tables give very similar results. In the case of Sweden, the life tables calculated were compared with the official life tables constructed from death and population statistics. These tables also show similar results.

[9]Actually, it is possible to assume that the population under 10 and over age 60 is zero and to obtain the same life table, as is explained in footnote 11 below.

census was taken--was made in the following manner. The 10-year age group distribution between ages 10 and 59 was smoothed and separated into 5-year age groups. The proportions of the 5-year age groups related to the total population were calculated, and then were divided by a particular $_5L_x$ value from the model life tables.[10] The natural logarithms of these quotients were adjusted to a straight line by least squares, and extrapolated to all ages (the slope of the straight line should be as close as possible to the natural growth rate of the country); then the antilogarithms of the adjusted values were taken and multiplied by the same set of $_5L_x$ from the model life tables. The result is assumed to be the proportional 5-year age distribution of the stable population under the demographic characteristics of the country at that particular date. The adjustment by the least square method allows us to calculate the intrinsic birth rate--b--by finding the ordinate of the origin, that is, C(0). C(0) is the proportion of persons at exact age zero in the stable population, that is, b.[11] With the previous information, the $_5L_x$ function of the life tables can be obtained by using the following equation:

$$_5L_x = \frac{1}{b} C(x, x + 4) e^{r(x + 2.5)}$$

From the $_5L_x$ the other functions of the life tables are easily found by the usual methods.

As mentioned above, the new life tables are more accurate than the previous ones, especially for the earliest dates. The differences between the new and previous life tables, which widen as one goes back in time, narrow in the 1960's. The earlier life tables give, in general, a lower mortality level. A comparison between the old and new life tables of all possible dates is presented in Table II-1. The smaller difference between the two tables in the period 1900-1929 in comparison with subsequent periods appears to be an exception, but actually it is not. The differences for 1900-1929 are of considerable magnitude because

---

[10] The models were those of the United Nations, Methods for Population Projections by Sex and Age, Manual III, ST/SOA/Series A, Population Studies No. 25 (New York, 1956). Details are explained in Arriaga, New Life Tables.

[11] If the actual population in ages under 10 and 60 and over is assumed to be zero, each proportion of the age groups between 10 and 59 will increase proportionately. The assumption will shift the adjusted straight line by the least squares method by a constant, affecting the intrinsic birth rate and the C(x,x+4) values in the same proportion. But because we divided the C(x,x+4) values by the intrinsic birth rate in order to obtain the $_5L_x$ function, this function is independent of such effect.

LATIN AMERICAN DATA USED

Table II-1

COMPARISON BETWEEN NEW AND PREVIOUS LIFE TABLES FOR LATIN AMERICA

		Average Life Expectancy at Birth (years)		
Period of Time[a]	Number of Comparisons	Previous Tables	New Tables	Percent Difference
Prior to 1900	2	31.1	25.5	22
1900-1929	7	31.6	29.8	6
1930-1949	12	42.9	37.1	16
Since 1950	33	53.2	51.2	4

[a]Countries in each period:

Prior to 1900: Brazil and Mexico
1900-1920: Brazil, Chile, and Mexico
1930-1949: Chile, Colombia, Mexico, and Venezuela
Since 1950: Bolivia, Brazil, Chile, Costa Rica, Dominican Republic, El Salvador, Guatemala, Haiti, Mexico, Panama, and Peru

Source: Arriaga and Davis, "Pattern of Mortality Change."

the comparison utilizes the Brazilian, Chilean, and Mexican life tables, the data of which even at that date were fairly good--at least more accurate than life tables for other countries. In the subsequent period, however, Brazil was not included, while Colombia and Venezuela--both with poor registration--were added. These two countries had incomplete death registration at that time; consequently, the life tables constructed with such data will overestimate the level of life expectancy--or underestimate the level of mortality. The differences between the life expectancies of the earlier and new life tables for these two countries are of such magnitude that the differences of all the countries compared in periods after 1929 became greater than in the previous period. If, however, the same countries are followed through time, from prior to 1900 to after 1929, the trend of life expectancies remains quite consistent. A previously cited study states:

Unfortunately, we do not have enough comparisons to be able to deal with the same group of countries throughout the four periods. However, there are three countries (Brazil, Chile, and Mexico) for which comparisons can be made at three or more dates. Grouping the tables into "early," "intermediate," and "recent" for each of them, we get the following comparisons:

	Number of Life Tables Compared	Average Life Expectancy		
		Previous Tables	Our Tables	Percent Difference
Early	10	29.8	27.1	9.7
Intermediate	12	38.2	35.4	6.5
Recent	10	52.6	51.4	2.3

The main reason for the generally lower life-expectancy in our life tables lies in the greater reliability of the information on which they are based. In previous life tables the varying degrees of completeness of the censuses and of the vital statistics were the principal source of error. In the case of Brazil, where no vital statistics were used and where the life tables were deduced from intercensal survival ratios, differential census completeness was the cause of error. This hypothesis not only explains why the differences in life-expectancy between the new life tables and the previously existing ones become greater as we go back in history, but it also accounts for the fact that the widest discrepancies occur at the young and the old ages.

If the previous and the new life tables are compared with respect to the probability of surviving a given number of years [see Table II-2 below], the differences by age appear clearly. For dates prior to 1960, the probability of surviving from age 0 to age 15 is 5 percent higher in previous life tables than in ours; the probability of surviving from age 45 to 70 is 14 percent higher; but the probability of lasting from age 15 to age 45 is only 2 percent higher.

The discrepancy at young ages is due to the usual fact of underregistration of infant deaths, which tends to reduce the probability of dying when the infant mortality is incorporated in the traditional life tables. In the older ages the discrepancy stems both from some failures in registration and, more

> commonly, from exaggeration of age by persons of advanced years. As a consequence of these two irregularities in vital statistics and census enumeration, the conventional life tables substantially overstate survivorship at both ends of life.[12]

As a consequence of the overestimation of life expectancy by previous life tables, the rapidity of mortality decline in these countries has been underestimated. In other words, the mortality decline has been faster than the trend shown by the previous life tables. The differences can be seen in Tables II-1 and II-2.

Table II-2

SURVIVAL RATIOS OF NEW AND PREVIOUS LIFE TABLES: BEFORE AND AFTER 1960

	$_{15}P_{0}$	$_{15}P_{15}$	$_{15}P_{30}$	$_{25}P_{45}$
For 23 tables before 1960:				
New	.693	.879	.832	.434
Previous	.726	.897	.847	.495
Percent difference	4.7	2.0	1.8	14.1
For 10 tables after 1960:				
New	.844	.952	.919	.606
Previous	.859	.961	.929	.659
Percent difference	1.8	.9	1.1	8.7

Source: Arriaga and Davis, "Pattern of Mortality Change," p. 225.

[12]Arriaga and Davis, "Pattern of Mortality Change," pp. 224-225.

The life expectancies at birth of the new life tables were taken as the best index for an international comparison of the general mortality level of these countries, which is made in the next chapter. The detailed analysis of the mortality decline by sex and age from 1930 to the 1960's has been based principally on the ${}_5L_x$ function of the abridged life tables (see Chapter IV). In Chapter V a particular method of analysis is used to detect the effect of the mortality decline on the age structure.

Fertility Information

Detailed fertility information for Latin America is not only scarce, but incomplete in the few available series. Primarily crude birth rates are used in this study, preferably those estimated by Collver.[13] Official crude birth rates, however, also are used in a few cases. In addition, births by age of mother for the 1960's are used to estimate age-specific fertility rates. The accuracy of the analysis rests on the trends discerned, rather than on the level of fertility. Fortunately, due to the use of excellent fertility estimates, both fertility trends and levels are close to actuality.

Conclusion

The new mortality information makes it possible for this study to deal with most of the larger countries of Latin America. Because of the characteristics of the new set of life tables, we are able to achieve a wider coverage of the area with more accurate information than has been possible in the past.

---

[13] Collver, Birth Rates.

P A R T II

THE MORTALITY DECLINE IN LATIN AMERICA

Chapter III

THE RAPID RISE OF LIFE EXPECTANCY

A few decades ago, in the 1930's, mortality was very high in most Latin American countries. Under the mortality conditions of that period, a newborn baby had less than a 50 percent chance of being alive at age 30. In general, there was no country with a life expectancy of over 40 years at birth. More recently, under mortality conditions of the 1960's, a newborn baby had more than a 50 percent chance of being alive at age 60. The life tables for these years show life expectancies of between 50 and 60 years at birth.[1] The purpose of this chapter is to establish the general mortality trend for most of the countries by using levels of life expectancy at birth.

The rapidly declining mortality trend in this area suggests the value of a comparison between the historical mortality trend in these countries and the European historical trend, and an examination of the factors producing the different trends. After establishing Latin American mortality trends, we shall compare them to European trends, establish any differences, and attempt to explain them. Three Latin American countries have not been included in this study because they lack historical mortality information: Argentina, Cuba, and Uruguay.[2]

Historical Mortality Trends in Latin America[3]

The available life tables show an extremely low life expectancy at birth for the whole area during the nineteenth century.[4] Excluding the three countries mentioned above--

---

[1] Arriaga, New Life Tables.

[2] The new method of life table construction was not applied to them because the populations of these countries could not be considered quasi-stable.

[3] This section closely follows the previous study by Arriaga and Davis, "Pattern of Mortality Change."

[4] The life tables used in this study have been taken from Arriaga, New Life Tables.

Argentina, Cuba, and Uruguay--it is possible to say that, before 1900, life expectancies at birth in Latin American countries fluctuated around 30 years and were increasing at a very slow pace. The period from 1900 to 1930, when mortality was declining faster than it had before 1900, was still one of slow mortality decline. The whole region added an average of only .21 years to the life expectancy at birth per annum. The situation changed completely after 1930, when mortality began declining sharply. The average gain in life expectancy at birth per annum was .74 years during 1930-1960 (see Table III-1).

Table III-1

CHANGES IN LIFE EXPECTANCY AT BIRTH IN LATIN AMERICA: 1860-1960

Period	Life Expectancy (years)		Annual Years Added	Annual Percent Change
	Starting	Ending		
1860-1870	24.4	25.0	.06	.25
1870-1880	25.0	25.5	.05	.20
1880-1890	25.5	26.1	.06	.24
1890-1900	26.1	27.2	.11	.42
1900-1910	27.2	28.9	.17	.63
1910-1920	28.9	31.1	.22	.76
1920-1930	31.1	33.6	.25	.80
1930-1940	33.6	38.0	.44	1.31
1940-1950	38.0	46.4	.84	2.21
1950-1960	46.4	55.8	.94	2.03
1860-1900	24.4	27.2	.09	.38
1900-1930	27.2	33.6	.21	.78
1930-1960	33.6	55.8	.74	2.20

Source: Arriaga and Davis, "Pattern of Mortality Change," pp. 223-242.

The historical trends for individual countries are not all similar. In some countries, the mortality decline not only started earlier than in others, but also proceeded at a faster pace. The mortality level differences among these countries changed continuously during the period from 1900 to 1960. (The mean, standard deviation, and coefficient of variation of the life expectancies at birth for each decade can be seen in Table III-2.) The coefficient of variation was .088 in 1900 and .087 in 1960; this means that at both dates these countries had almost the same relative differences in life expectancy. During the 60 years between the two dates, however, the coefficients of variation fluctuated considerably: they increased to a peak of .132 in 1930, and then declined to close to the initial level (see Table III-2).

At the end of the past century and the beginning of the present, countries such as Chile, Colombia, Brazil, Costa Rica, Mexico, and Panama had a lower mortality than countries such as the Dominican Republic, Guatemala, and Nicaragua. (For simplicity, the first group of countries are labeled Group A and the second, Group B.) Between 1900 and 1930, the Group A countries not only had a lower mortality level, but also a faster rate of mortality decline than the countries of Group B, as can be seen from the changes in life expectancies given in Table III-3. During the second period, 1930 to 1960, the reduction in mortality in the whole area was extremely rapid and progressed at almost the same rate in all countries. For instance, the average life expectancy at birth in the two groups of countries remained at almost the same absolute difference--7 to 9 years--after 1930, a fact reflected in the same number of years added annually to the life expectancies at birth in each group (see Figure III-1). An explanation of why this particular difference has existed between the two groups of Latin American countries follows.

Table III-2

MORTALITY DIFFERENCES AMONG LATIN AMERICAN COUNTRIES: 1900-1960

	1900	1910	1920	1930	1940	1950	1960
Number of countries	7	8	9	14	15	17	14
Mean life expectancy	27.2	29.1	30.8	32.9	38.0	45.7	55.1
Standard deviation	2.38	2.58	3.28	4.35	4.17	4.80	4.78
Coefficient of variation	.088	.089	.106	.132	.110	.105	.087

Source: Arriaga and Davis, "Pattern of Mortality Change," pp. 223-242.

Table III-3

LIFE EXPECTANCIES AT BIRTH IN TWO GROUPS OF LATIN AMERICAN COUNTRIES: 1860-1960

	Life Expectancy (years)		Differences		Annual Years Added To Life Expectancy Per Decade	
			Absolute	Percent		
	Group A[a]	Group B[b]	(1)-(2)	(3):(2)	Group A	Group B
Year	(1)	(2)	(3)	(4)	(5)	(6)
1860	25.1					
1870	25.9				.08	
1880	26.6				.07	
1890	27.2	23.4	3.8	16.2	.06	
1900	28.5	23.9	4.6	19.2	.13	.05
1910	30.5	24.6	5.9	24.0	.20	.07
1920	33.0	25.3	7.7	30.4	.25	.07
1930	36.1	27.1	9.0	33.2	.31	.18
1940	40.2	33.0	7.2	21.8	.41	.59
1950	48.9	40.7	8.2	20.1	.87	.77
1960	58.2	50.4	7.8	15.5	.93	.97

[a] Group A countries: Brazil, Chile, Colombia, Costa Rica, Mexico, and Panama.

[b] Group B countries: Dominican Republic, Guatemala, and Nicaragua.

Source: Arriaga and Davis, "Pattern of Mortality Change, pp. 223-242.

Figure III-1

HISTORICAL TRENDS IN LIFE EXPECTANCY IN LATIN AMERICA: 1860-1960

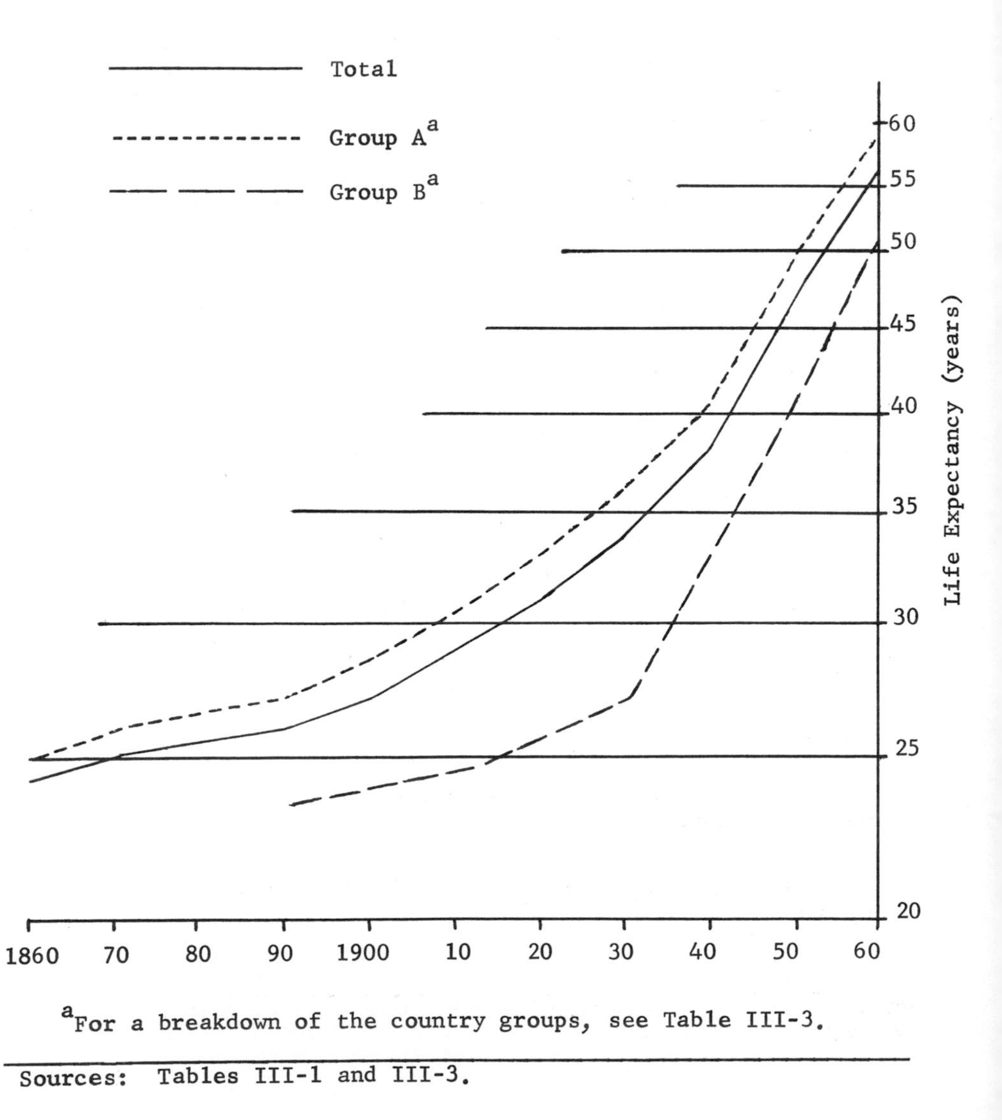

[a]For a breakdown of the country groups, see Table III-3.

Sources: Tables III-1 and III-3.

Differential Mortality Trends Among Latin American Countries. Two interesting facts emerge from Table III-1. First, a noticeable mortality decline started in Group A countries after 1910, a decline that was even more rapid after 1930. Second, Group B countries had a very slow mortality decline before 1930 and a very rapid one after that date.

Before the 1930's, the mortality condition in Group A countries was not only better than that in Group B countries, but also its decline was faster. The mortality trends in these two groups of countries fit perfectly into the theory of changes in mortality in modern times, which maintains that the decline of mortality--principally from high levels--is related to improvements in a society's living conditions and economic situation.[5] If this is the case, mortality can be taken as an index of the stage of economic development of the population.[6] For instance, if mortality is very high--in other words, if life expectancy is very low--we would expect a country's living and economic conditions to be at a primitive stage and the reduction of mortality almost nil until the situation changed. This was precisely the situation in the Group B countries up to 1930. On the other hand, Group A countries, which in 1910 had a life expectancy at birth of over 30 years, raised their life expectancy in the next 20 years quite rapidly. In Latin America in the two decades following 1910, the higher the level of life expectancy at birth, the faster its rate of change (see Table III-3). This would seem to indicate that the mortality decline in the region until the 1930's was directly connected with the improvement of living conditions resulting from better economic circumstances.

Although the above argument holds prior to 1930, after that date it is no longer valid. Since 1930, both Groups A and

---

[5]Probably the best example is provided by England and Wales during the period from 1850 to the end of the nineteenth century. See McKeown and Record, "Declining of Mortality in England and Wales."

[6]At least it is not to be expected that if a country's economic level is high, mortality is high. People in some countries in the past, however--for instance, whites in New Zealand and Australia--have had relatively high life expectancies before the country developed. In other words, mortality was relatively lower than it should have been when related to the economic condition of the country. But it should be remembered that these two countries received a great many immigrants from European countries--principally England--and that although the countries were not economically developed, the society was.
See also Arriaga and Davis, "Pattern of Mortality Change."

B have registered a similar and very rapid increase of life expectancy at birth, regardless of the mortality level already reached. The mortality level and its change--principally the latter--can no longer be seen as dependent upon economic development. There is no doubt that other factors are at work. Among them, probably the most important is the improvement of public health facilities and medical care.

Some comparisons between Latin American and European historical mortality trends will help explain why all Latin American countries had such a similar mortality decline after 1930.

Comparison of Latin American and European Mortality Declines

Europe has been chosen for purposes of comparison because several countries there possess extensive (over time) economic and demographic data. In addition, the economic development of certain Eastern European countries has been delayed in relation to Western European countries. The comparison of different economic and demographic patterns of development will reveal not only the distinctions between the Latin American and European mortality declines, but also the reasons for the dissimilarity.

For the purpose of analysis, it is useful to divide European countries into two groups. The first group contains those early industrialized nations in which mortality in Europe was always at its lowest level--at least since the middle of the nineteenth century, when data series began. Denmark, England and Wales, France, Holland, Norway, Scotland, Sweden, and Switzerland will be designated Group 1. The rest of Europe--that is, those countries which industrialized later than those in Group 1--will be called Group 2.[7] In the comparison of mortality in the European countries and Latin America, the life expectancy at birth will be used, as before, as a measure of the general mortality level.[8]

---

[7]Germany is not included because at the beginning of the comparison period (1860) it was like a Group 2 country and at the end of the period like a Group 1 country.

[8]The life expectancy data for Europe are taken from Robert Kuczynski, The Measurement of Population Growth (London: Sidwick and Jackson Ltd., 1935) and The Balance of Births and Deaths (Vol. I--New York: The MacMillan Co., 1928, and Vol. II--Washington, D.C.: The Brookings Institution, 1931); Coghill C. Case, J. Harley, and J. Pearson, The Chester Beatty Research Institute, Serial Abridged Life Tables, 1841-1960 (London: The Chester

In the 1860's, the average life expectancy for the Group 1 countries in Europe was 40.7 years, while for Latin America as a whole it was 24.4 years--a difference of 16.3 years. One hundred years later, in the 1960's, the life expectancies of the two regions were 71.8 and 55.8 years, respectively--a difference of 16.0 years (Table III-4). Apparently, judging from these two points of reference, the discrepancy between the mortality levels of the two areas remained constant during the period. This was not the case, however. During this 100-year period, the two regions exhibited quite different patterns of mortality decline, as seen in Figure III-2 and Table III-4. The differences between the life expectancies of Latin American and European countries increased until the 1930's due to the faster mortality decline in Group 1 countries in Europe. After that, the faster mortality decline in Latin America than in Europe reduced the mortality difference of the two areas until they approached--perhaps randomly--almost the same difference in life expectancies at birth as at the beginning of the period considered. Of course, a difference of 16 years between life expectancies at birth when the lesser life expectancy is 55 years is relatively less than when the lesser life expectancy is 24 years. Latin American mortality, compared to the mortality of Group 1, was in a much better position in 1960 than in 1860.

The life expectancy growth rates[9] for the Group 1 European countries remained almost constant during the 100-year period. The decade rates changed smoothly; they approached a plane-shaped curve (Table III-5 and Figure III-3).

On the other hand, the life expectancy growth rates in Latin American countries increased during the whole period. Thus, the changing differences between the life expectancies in the two groups of countries can be attributed to the changing pace of mortality in Latin America. In 1860, the mortality decline in these countries was slower than in the Group 1 European countries; between 1890 and 1930 the decline was almost the same in both groups; after the 1930's the mortality decline was much faster in Latin America than in the Group 1 countries, as seen in Table III-5. (Absolute and relative differences in life expectancies at birth between both groups of countries can be seen in Table III-4.)

Beatty Research Institute, Institute of Cancer Research, Royal Cancer Hospital, 1962); Statistiska Centralbyran, Statistisk Arsbok (several years) and Historisk Statistik für Sverige (1720-1950) (Stockholm, 1955).

[9]These rates are the annual average geometric growth rates of the life expectancies during each decade, per thousand.

Table III-4

LIFE EXPECTANCIES AT BIRTH IN TWO GROUPS OF EUROPEAN COUNTRIES AND LATIN AMERICA: 1860-1960

	Life Expectancies at Birth (years)			Differences			
	Europe		Latin America	Absolute		Percents	
Years	Group 1[a]	Group 2[b]		(1)-(3)	(2)-(3)	(4):(3)	(5):(3)
	(1)	(2)	(3)	(4)	(5)	(6)	(7)
1860	40.7	26.4	24.4	16.3	2.0	66.8	8.2
1870	41.5	27.5	25.0	16.5	2.5	66.0	10.0
1880	43.3	30.0	25.5	17.8	4.5	69.8	17.6
1890	45.4	32.1	26.1	19.3	6.0	73.9	23.0
1900	47.8	35.0	27.2	20.6	7.8	75.7	28.7
1910	50.8	39.9	28.9	21.9	11.0	75.8	38.1
1920	55.0	46.1	31.1	23.9	15.0	76.8	48.2
1930	59.9	50.9	33.6	26.3	17.3	78.3	51.5
1940	64.8	56.0	38.0	26.8	18.0	70.5	47.3
1950	68.8	63.4	46.4	22.4	17.0	48.3	36.6
1960	71.8	68.0	55.8	16.0	12.2	28.7	21.9

[a]Group 1 countries: Denmark, England and Wales, France, Holland, Norway, Scotland, Sweden, and Switzerland.

[b]Group 2 countries: Rest of Europe, excluding Germany.

Sources: Latin America: Arriaga and Davis, "Pattern of Mortality Change," pp. 223-242; Europe: Calculated from the information given by Kuczynski in Measurement of Population Growth and Balance of Births and Deaths.

RAPID RISE OF LIFE EXPECTANCY

Figure III-2

HISTORICAL TRENDS IN LIFE EXPECTANCY IN EUROPEAN COUNTRY GROUPS AND LATIN AMERICA: 1860-1960

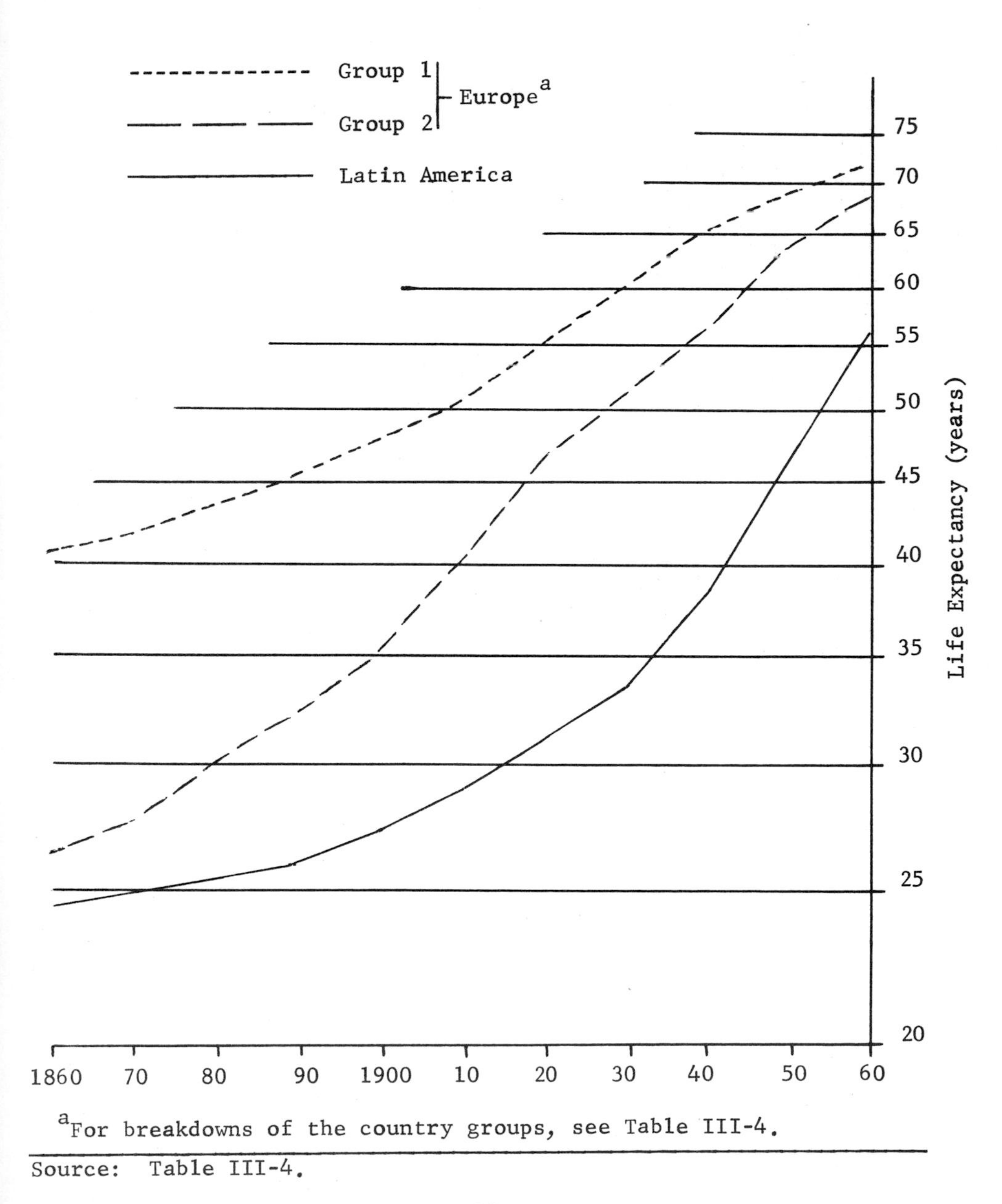

[a]For breakdowns of the country groups, see Table III-4.

Source: Table III-4.

Table III-5

ANNUAL LIFE EXPECTANCY GROWTH RATES FOR EUROPEAN AND LATIN AMERICAN COUNTRY GROUPS: 1850-1960

	Actual Rates[a]					Smoothed Rates[a]				
	Latin America			Europe		Latin America			Europe	
Period	Total	Group A[b]	Group B[c]	Group 1[d]	Group 2[e]	Total	Group A	Group B	Group 1	Group 2
1850-1860	--	--	--	1.5	3.1	--	--	--	1.5	3.1
1860-1870	2.4	3.1	--	1.9	4.1	2.4	3.1	--	2.4	5.0
1870-1880	2.0	2.7	--	4.2	8.7	2.2	2.7	--	3.8	7.1
1880-1890	2.3	2.2	--	4.7	6.8	2.7	3.0	--	4.7	7.7
1890-1900	4.1	4.7	2.1	5.2	8.6	4.2	4.6	2.1	5.3	9.3
1900-1910	6.4	6.8	2.9	6.1	13.1	6.1	6.6	2.7	6.3	12.3
1910-1920	7.3	7.9	2.8	7.9	14.4	7.2	7.9	3.9	7.6	13.0
1920-1930	7.7	9.0	6.9	8.5	9.9	8.8	9.2	9.1	8.2	10.9
1930-1940	12.3	10.8	19.7	7.9	9.5	13.1	12.6	16.8	7.6	10.3
1940-1950	20.0	19.6	21.0	6.0	12.4	17.7	16.7	20.8	6.1	10.3
1950-1960	18.4	17.4	21.4	4.3	7.0	18.4	17.4	21.4	4.3	7.0

[a] These rates are the annual average geometric growth rates for each decade, per thousand.

[b] Group A: Brazil, Chile, Colombia, Costa Rica, Mexico, and Panama.

[c] Group B: Dominican Republic, Nicaragua, and Guatemala.

[d] Group 1: Denmark, England and Wales, France, Holland, Norway, Scotland, Sweden, and Switzerland.

[e] Group 2: Rest of Europe, excluding Germany.

Source: Calculated from Tables III-3 and III-4.

Figure III-3

LIFE EXPECTANCY GROWTH RATES FOR EUROPEAN AND LATIN AMERICAN COUNTRY GROUPS

(Smoothed Rates)

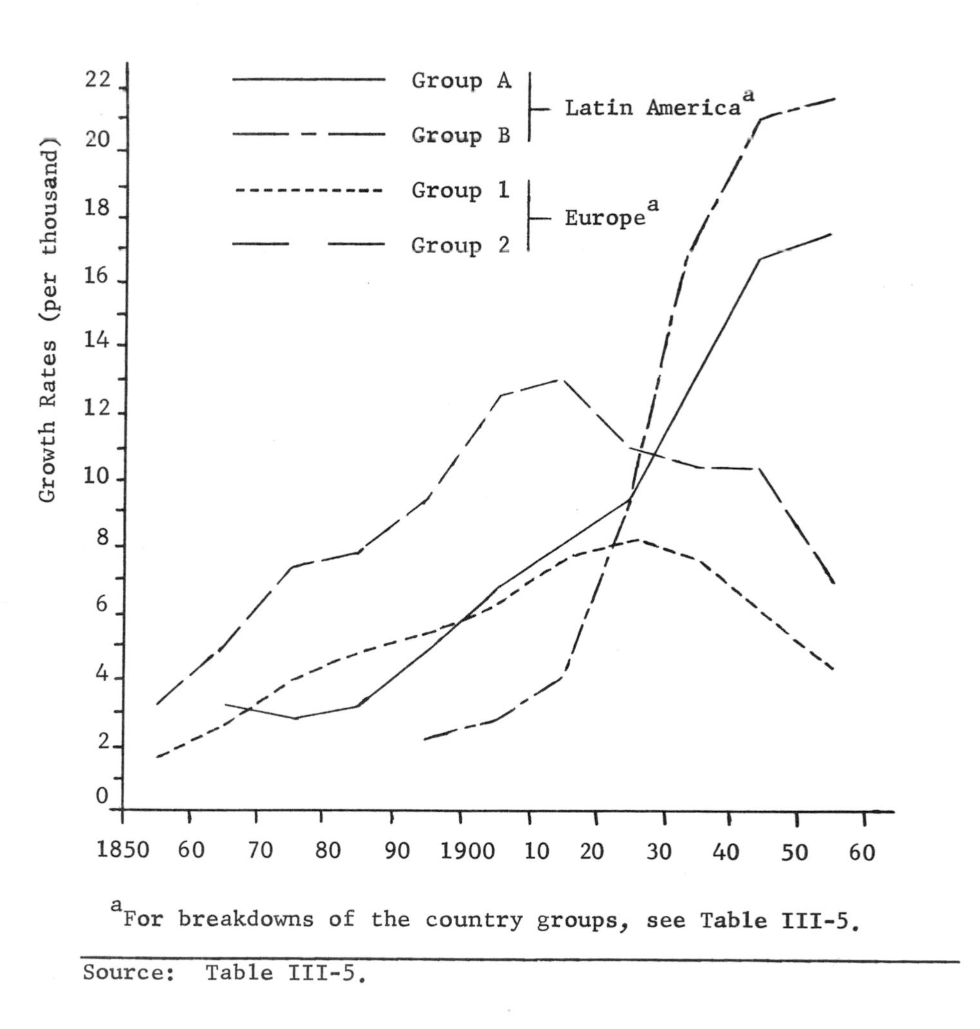

[a]For breakdowns of the country groups, see Table III-5.

Source: Table III-5.

The comparison of Latin American countries with the Group 2 European countries resembles the previous comparison, although a difference occurs in the first part of the 100-year period. In the 1860's the Group 2 countries had a life expectancy at birth which was close to that of the Latin American countries--only two years longer (26.3 and 24.4 years, respectively).[10] At the end of the period, in 1960, the Group 2 countries had a life expectancy 12 years longer than the Latin American countries--68.0 and 55.8 years, respectively (Table III-4). The life expectancy growth rates for the Group 2 countries take the same shape as those of Group 1, but are more leptokurtic (Table III-5 and Figure III-3). The life expectancy differences between the Group 2 countries and Latin America were at a maximum around 1930. After that year the decline in Latin America was more rapid than in the Group 2 countries; however, a difference of 12.2 years between the life expectancies was observed in 1960 (Figure III-2). Almost the same results are obtained if, instead of the whole of Latin America, Group A is compared with European Groups 1 and 2 (Tables III-3, III-4, and III-5).

The pattern of mortality decline in Latin America differs from that of Europe principally in the rate of decline (from a given mortality level) and the period when decline occurred. Let us now consider why the two patterns were different.

The Relation of Mortality Decline to Economic Conditions and Public Health

Because mortality is directly or indirectly related to economic conditions and public health, it is possible to write symbolically that

$$M = F(EC, PH).$$

The relationship between mortality (M), economic conditions (EC), and public health (PH) in the early industrial countries was different from that in a currently developing country. In the European Group 1 countries, for example, public health programs were a direct reflection of economic conditions. (By public health programs, I refer not only to the improvement of nutrition and living conditions for the population, but also to the development of improved medical equipment, research institutions, etc.) Since advances in public health depended primarily on the speed of economic development in these countries, and mortality rate changes reflected advances in public health, we may say that

[10] The mortality decline in the Group 2 countries started later than in the Group 1 countries.

mortality levels in the early industrial countries in Europe depended directly on the economic condition of each country, with other factors having little practical importance. As the economies of the countries improved step by step, mortality decline progressed in a like manner.

Public health programs in currently backward countries, on the contrary, are not so dependent upon the countries' economic development. These countries do not have to develop and maintain a major medical establishment of their own; rather, they can "import" new techniques, discoveries, or drugs from more advanced nations, as well as receive international financial or material aid. Hence the public health variable is almost independent of the country's economy; it depends a great deal on medical progress and development in *other* countries. In other words--assuming that most new medical discoveries occur in the most economically advanced countries--the public health program of an underdeveloped country is related more to the economy of the advanced countries than it is to its own economy. Therefore, with respect to mortality, the economic variable in a backward country has lost importance, while the public health variable has come to have greater weight.

In order to understand the mortality behavior of the regions considered here, another point must be kept in mind: progress in medical science not only depends on material factors (equipment, capital, professional workers, etc.), but is also influenced by a time factor. Since the world keeps scientific records, more and more knowledge is constantly accumulated; thus current medical practice is more effective than that of a hundred years ago. Medical knowledge is available to any country, developed or underdeveloped. Hence, because public health programs in backward countries depend largely on other countries, we can expect that *the later in historical time a massive public health program is applied in an underdeveloped country previously lacking public health programs, the higher the rate of mortality decline will be*.

This assertion is ideally illustrated in Figure III-4, where four groups of countries--Latin American Groups A and B, European Groups 1 and 2--have been plotted. The upper line (Group 1 countries) has a smaller slope (signifying a slower rate of change) than the others. Mortality rates were contingent on public health programs, which advanced as economic development proceeded. The countries of Group 2 were less developed than those of Group 1 at the end of the past century and had a higher mortality rate than the latter. However, because of geographical proximity and good communications between Group 1 and Group 2 countries, medical knowledge and discoveries quickly spread to Group 2 countries, even before the latter started economic development. After 1900, Group 2 countries rapidly reduced the

Figure III-4

HISTORICAL TRENDS IN LIFE EXPECTANCIES IN EUROPEAN AND LATIN AMERICAN COUNTRY GROUPS

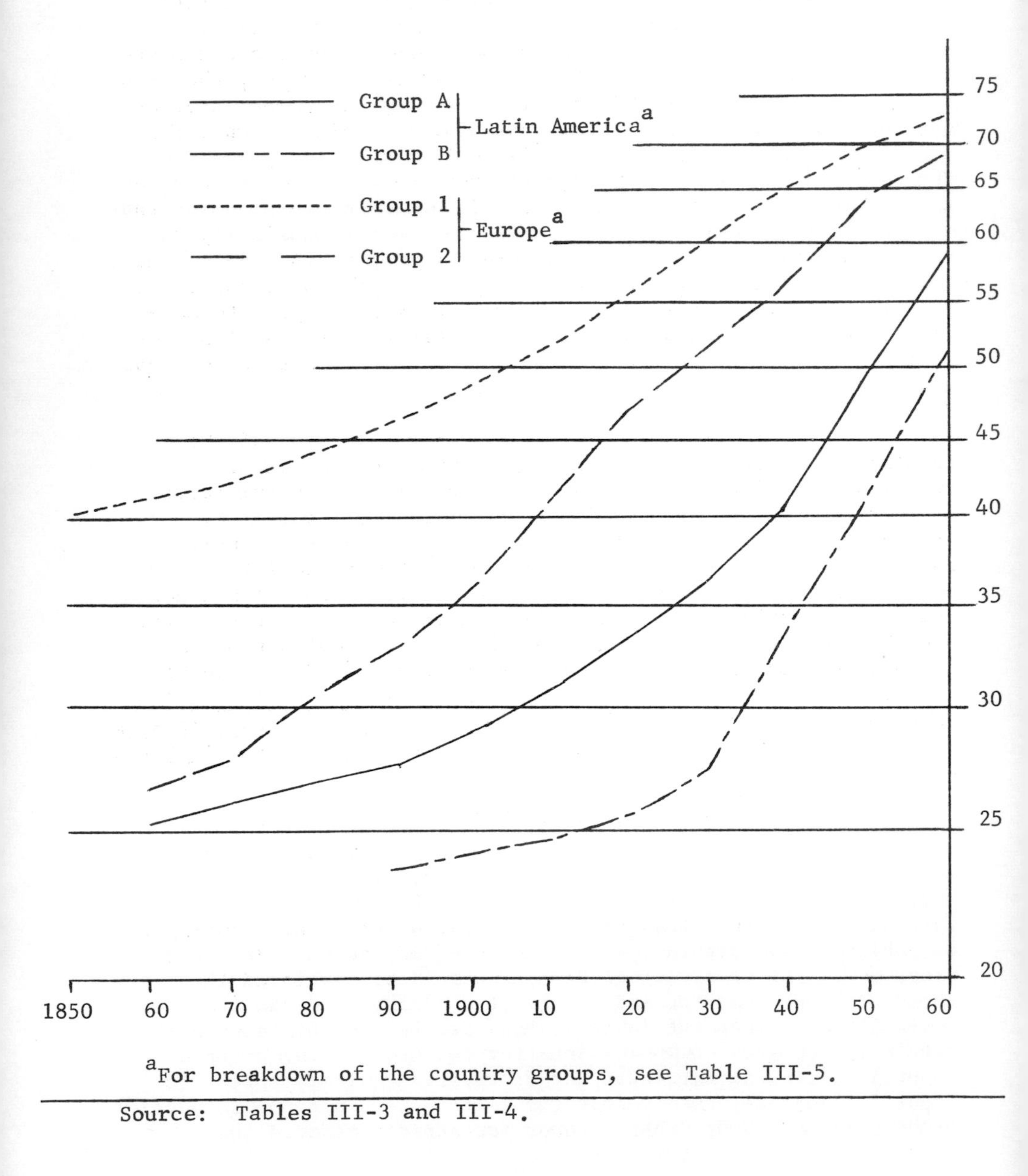

[a]For breakdown of the country groups, see Table III-5.

Source: Tables III-3 and III-4.

difference between the two average life expectancies of the European groups. The gap of 14.4 years in 1860 was reduced to 3.8 years in 1960.

Group A Latin American countries had a slow mortality decline before 1900. From 1900 to 1930 we may conjecture that they were improving living conditions as a consequence of a probable improvement in their economy, but at the same time--with a lag of some years compared to European Group 2 countries--some "imported" public health measures were applied. Since 1930 Group A nations have increased these "imports" and have also benefitted from international public health programs.

The Group B Latin American countries have only more recently begun to "import" medical help. They have experienced the most rapid mortality decline over time--even greater than Group A countries (see Table III-5 and Figure III-3).

In a population the change from high to low mortality is principally due to the reduction of infectious-communicable diseases.[11] In currently developing countries, the reduction of infectious-communicable diseases can be achieved in a short period of time.[12] As a previous study points out:

> At the present, regardless of the stage of development of a country, certain public health and medical techniques can be applied--principally those measures whose applications are not expensive. These include community health measures such as eradication of disease vectors, chlorination of drinking water, and good sewage systems, as well as individual health practices such as vaccination, dietary supplements, use of new drugs, and better personal hygiene. These techniques need not necessarily have been developed locally since they can be imported. As a consequence, a backward country can succeed in combating a particular infectious-communicable disease without having to develop or maintain a major medical establishment of its own.[13]

---

[11] Arriaga, "Rural-Urban Mortality in Developing Countries."

[12] Public health programs are first applied in cities. Data for the adult population (different results would appear if the total population were considered) living in eleven large Latin American cities show a very low level of deaths due to infectious-communicable diseases in the 1960's. See R.R. Puffer and W.G. Griffith, Patterns of Urban Mortality (Washington, D.C.: Pan American Health Organization, Sept. 1967).

[13] Arriaga and Davis, "Pattern of Mortality Decline."

Interesting examples of rapid mortality decline are to be found in Venezuela in Latin America, Russia in Europe, and Ceylon and Japan in Asia. It would be difficult to explain the mortality decline that these countries have experienced solely in terms of economic prosperity. In the case of Russia, medical knowledge and techniques were learned, to some extent, from other more advanced countries during the years after the Bolshevik revolution. Russian scientists did not need to rediscover the medical knowledge circulating in Western Europe; they did not have to suffer a lengthy apprenticeship in research, discovery, and testing. Medical developments and information brought in from other countries allowed the Soviets to produce disease-combating drugs almost immediately.

The rapid mortality decline in Japan paralleled that in Russia.[14] The aid that Ceylon received in public health programs is well known, as is the rapid mortality decline.[15]

---

[14]For data on the Japanese mortality decline, see Irene B. Taeuber, The Population of Japan (Princeton, N.J.: Princeton University Press, 1958), pp. 284-309.

[15]The mortality decline in Ceylon has been the source of some controversy. The eradication of malaria has been cited as the principal cause (see Population Reference Bureau, Inc., Worldwide War on Malaria [Washington, D.C.: Population Bulletin, March, 1958] and P.F. Russell, Man's Mastery of Malaria [Oxford University Press, 1955]), but there has not been a unanimous consensus on this point. Harald Frederiksen asserts in two articles that "the available evidence fails to establish malaria control as the sole or major cause of population explosion in Ceylon." (Frederiksen attributes the population explosion to falling mortality, with fertility remaining high. See Harald Frederiksen, "Malaria Control and Population Pressure in Ceylon," Public Health Reports 75, No. 10 [October 1960] and "Determinants and Consequences of Mortality Trends in Ceylon," Public Health Reports 76, No. 8 [August 1961]).

Whether the eradication of malaria in Ceylon was the principal cause of mortality decline can in truth be argued. But the fact remains that malaria control together with several other measures did reduce mortality in the country. Ceylon not only directly benefitted from malaria control and other public health measures--such as "imported" medical knowledge, techniques, equipment, and drugs--but also indirectly benefitted from the eradication of malaria, which contributed to the reduction of death from other causes. Because of the eradication of malaria in rich agricultural areas, the possibility increased of improving nutrition, which plays an important role in successfully combatting other diseases.

The effect of imported public health programs in Venezuela is even better known. From 1936 to 1961 life expectancy increased at an average rate of 1.16 years per annum (from 33.9 to 62.9 years). Income from Venezuela's oil exports not only permitted an introduction of advanced medical knowledge from other countries, but it also brought international help in the eradication of vectors of certain communicable diseases.

It is now possible to explain the differences between the historical mortality trends in Latin America and Europe. The disparity in the patterns is due to the fact that after about 1930 public health programs in Latin America no longer depended on the economic level of the country, but rather on help from the more advanced countries in the world. Before 1930, it could be assumed that the level of mortality of any country reflected that country's economic situation; after that date, such an assumption was no longer applicable.

Summary

The historical mortality decline in Latin America can be divided into three different periods. Before 1900, mortality was not only at a very high level, but it remained almost constant over time as well. During the next 30 years, some countries (probably those with improved economic conditions) began to reduce mortality at a reasonable rate, while in others (presumably the less advanced countries) the decline was much slower. In the 1930's, the situation suddenly changed. All Latin American countries experienced a very rapid decline in mortality regardless of their levels of economic development. Since then, the mortality level no longer seems to be closely related to the economy of the country.

At least in Latin America, the speed of mortality decline seems to follow a general pattern: the later the date of decline, the faster its rate. Nationwide programs sponsored by each country and/or by international aid programs are the principal cause of this "rule." Public health programs are no longer dependent on the country's economy but rather, to a large degree, on the technology and concern of the most advanced countries in the world.

Chapter IV

THE PATTERN OF MORTALITY DECLINE BY AGE AND SEX

In the previous chapter we saw that the most rapid decline in Latin American mortality was observed from 1930 to 1960, when all of the countries reduced their mortality at an unprecedented rate for an area of such extensive size. In this chapter we shall concentrate on the changes the amazing mortality decline produced during this time in two other demographic parameters--the age structure and the sex distribution of the population.

Countries and Period To Be Covered

The period from 1930 to 1960 is, fortunately, the one with the most information available. This chapter deals with eleven Latin American countries having life tables both in or before the 1930's and in the 1960's--namely, Brazil, Chile, Costa Rica, El Salvador, Guatemala, Honduras, Mexico, Nicaragua, Panama, Paraguay, and Venezuela.[1]

In general, censuses in Latin American countries have not been taken regularly each decade. Therefore, the life tables do not cover exact 30-year periods, as would be most desirable for a comparative analysis of these countries. In order to render the periods comparable, an interpolation of the available life tables was made--the interpolated function being ${}_5L_x$. Two possibilities existed: either interpolate the nearest life tables in the 1960's and 1930's in order to have all values for 1960 and 1930, or interpolate only the life tables around 1930 to dates exactly 30 years earlier than the life tables for the 1960's. The second alternative (which requires the use of different calendar years for different countries) was adopted because of the

---

[1]The excluded countries are Bolivia and Colombia, which lack life tables for the 1960's; Dominican Republic, Ecuador, and Peru, which lack life tables for the 1930's or before; and Haiti, which lacks both.

If Argentina, Cuba, and Uruguay are excluded from the total (see Chapter II, footnote 2, above), the percent of the Latin American population included in the eleven countries was 75 percent in 1930 and 77 percent in 1960. It would be 62 percent and 66 percent, respectively, if these three countries were included in the total.

desire to retain accurate life tables for the 1960's. Furthermore, the possibility of obtaining a better interpolation is greater in the 1930's than in the 1960's because the differences of the pivotal values, between which the interpolation for the 1930's will fall, are smaller than in the 1960's, due to the slower mortality decline in earlier years.

A polynomial function was used in the interpolation for most countries. In Venezuela an exponential function was used for the interpolation between 1926 and 1936 (see Appendix IV), while for Chile, Mexico, and Panama an interpolation was not made because these countries already had life tables with exact 30-year intervals.

Indices Used

For the purposes of this study, we will use the change in the number of years lived by a population rather than the number of deaths saved as our index of mortality improvement. The number of years to be lived is measured by the L_x function of the life table. This function can be interpreted as the number of years to be lived between age x and x + 1 by those who were born at the same moment of time--that is, the radix of the table or the l_o--under constant mortality conditions. By using the cumulative number of years to be lived from age x up to the end of life (age ω), that is,

$$T_x = \sum_{i=0}^{\omega} L_{x+i},$$

and the number of persons alive at exact age $x(l_x)$, it is possible to define the temporary life expectancy at age x as:[2]

$$/n\ e_x = \frac{T_x - T_{x+n}}{l_x} \qquad \text{(IV-1)}$$

This formula gives the average number of years to be lived between ages x and x+n, under constant life table mortality conditions, by those who were alive at exact age x. (See detailed explanation in Appendix IV, pages 59-65 below.)

In order to measure the change in the number of years to be lived by each age group when mortality changes, two new indices

[2]José González Galé, Matemáticas Financieras (Segunda Parte), Elementos de Cálculo Actuarial (Buenos Aires: Librería El Ateneo Editorial, 1951).

have been used. The first is called the absolute change (${}_nAC_x$), which is simply the difference between the two temporary life expectancies for the same age groups, but under different mortality conditions. If the life tables, in which the mortality conditions of the population are reflected, were constructed in the years t and t+i, the absolute change index would be:

$${}_nAC_x^{t,t+i} = /n\ e_x^{t+i} - /n\ e_x^t \qquad \text{(IV-2)}$$

where the superscript refers to the year. The index ${}_nAC_x^{t,t+i}$ measures the change in the average number of years to be lived between ages x and x+n for those l_x persons alive at exact age x, due to the change in mortality between the years t and t+i.

The value of ${}_nAC_x^{t,t+i}$ depends on the level of life expectancy that has already been reached at the time t by the $/n\ e_x^t$, which cannot be greater than n. In other words, if the difference between n and $/n\ e_x^t$ is large, the value of ${}_nAC_x^{t,t+i}$ can also be large; but the value is small when the difference is small.

Another index to be used is the relative change index: ${}_nRC_x^{t,t+i}$. This index shows the increase in the average number of years to be lived between age x and x+n by those alive at exact age x in relation to the "possible" increase. In symbols,

$${}_nRC_x^{t,t+i} = \frac{{}_nAC_x^{t,t+i}}{n - /n\ e_x^t} \qquad \text{(IV-3)}$$

The relative change index ${}_nRC_x^{t,t+i}$ can also be considered as a measurement of the "effort" made to increase the average number of years to be lived between ages x and x+n for those alive at exact age x.

As in the case of other mortality indices, when the mortality effect is analyzed by age groups, the length of the age group--n--should remain constant for a better comparison.

The two indices shown above have been given for only one age x. The same indices can be applied for a group of two or more persons at the same or different ages x, y,...z. Later, these indices will be used for ages x and y in order to analyze the change in the number of years to be lived by a couple, where the man and woman are y and x years old respectively, for the purpose of relating the mortality decline to reproductive behavior. (See formulae and numerical examples in Appendix IV.)

Mortality Decline by Age

The magnitude of the mortality decline in Latin America differs with age. The mortality change by age depends not only upon the mortality level already reached in each particular age, but also upon the particular causes of death operating in each age.

In this part of the study, we shall analyze the age mortality decline by using the two indices previously described to establish the ages where the mortality decline was most significant. For this purpose, the calculation of the indices for 15-year age groups will be sufficient to give a general overview of the mortality changes by age, while for certain details, the indices calculated for 5-year age groups will be necessary.

The average of the absolute change index (${}_nAC_x^{t,t+i}$) for the eleven Latin American countries being considered shows clearly that the ages which benefitted most from mortality decline were those of childhood (see Table IV-1). Generally, under mortality conditions of the 1930's, a newborn baby lived only 10.1 years of the possible 15 from birth to age 15. Thirty years later, under mortality conditions of the 1960's, a newborn baby lived an average of 12.7 years of the possible 15--an increase of 2.6 years, or an average gain of more than one month per year between the two dates. Ages 15 to 30 benefitted least from the mortality decline. The 15-year temporary life expectancy of those alive at exact age 15 increased only .8 years under the changed mortality conditions from 1930 to 1960. The benefit received by each age group after 30 increased with age. The same pattern is repeated for each of the countries. (For details by country, see Appendix IV, Table A-IV-1.)

The average of the relative change index--the increase in the number of years to be lived in relation to the possible maximum increase between two ages because of the mortality decline--presents almost the opposite pattern of the absolute change, or more accurately, a "mirror-reflection" (see Figure IV-1). The values of the ${}_nRC_x$ index tell us that ages 15 to 30 were those which had the largest relative increase. This indicates that it was relatively easier to save lives in this age span than in others, assuming that equal efforts were made in all ages. The opposite is true in ages 60 to 74--the oldest group analyzed here--which had the smallest relative increase in the number of years to be lived.

Table IV-1

TEMPORARY LIFE EXPECTANCIES FOR 15-YEAR AGE GROUPS IN LATIN AMERICA: ABSOLUTE AND RELATIVE CHANGES, BOTH SEXES, 1930's TO 1960's

(Averages for eleven Latin American countries)[a]

		Age				
Index	Year(s)	0-14	15-29	30-44	45-59	60-74
$/n\ e_x$	1930	10.1432	13.9129	13.3233	12.3725	9.9345
$/n\ e_x$	1960	12.7475	14.6677	14.4441	13.8718	11.8985
${}_nAC_x$	1930-60	2.6043	.7548	1.1208	1.4993	1.9640
${}_nRC_x$	1930-60	.5362	.6943	.6685	.5706	.3877

[a]The countries are Brazil, Chile, Costa Rica, El Salvador, Guatemala, Honduras, Mexico, Nicaragua, Panama, Paraguay, and Venezuela.

Source: Appendix IV, Table A-IV-1.

Although the same pattern change seen in the 15-year age groups is found in the 5-year age groups, this last grouping allows us to establish with more accuracy those ages which received the maximum and minimum benefits from the mortality decline. The largest absolute increase in the number of years to be lived was registered in the ages under 5 (an average increase of .7 years between ages 0 to 5); the smallest by those in ages 10 to 14 (.07 years). From age 15, the gains increased continuously to the oldest ages (see Table IV-2). On the other hand, the largest relative increase was between ages 5 and 14, while the smallest was in the oldest age group, 80 to 84. As is the case for 15-year age groups, the trends of the indices ${}_nAC_x$ and ${}_nRC_x$ mirror each other (see Figure IV-1).

We saw in Chapter III that the mortality decline in Latin America since 1930 has been accelerated because of the countries' access to "imported" sanitary and medical knowledge. The mortality decline has been so rapid that the population cohorts at young adult ages (around 20 years old) in the 1930's increased their chances for survival as they grew older--a paradoxical

Figure IV-1

ABSOLUTE AND RELATIVE CHANGES IN THE NUMBER OF YEARS TO BE LIVED BECAUSE OF MORTALITY DECLINE BY 5- AND 15-YEAR AGE GROUPS IN LATIN AMERICA: 1930-1960

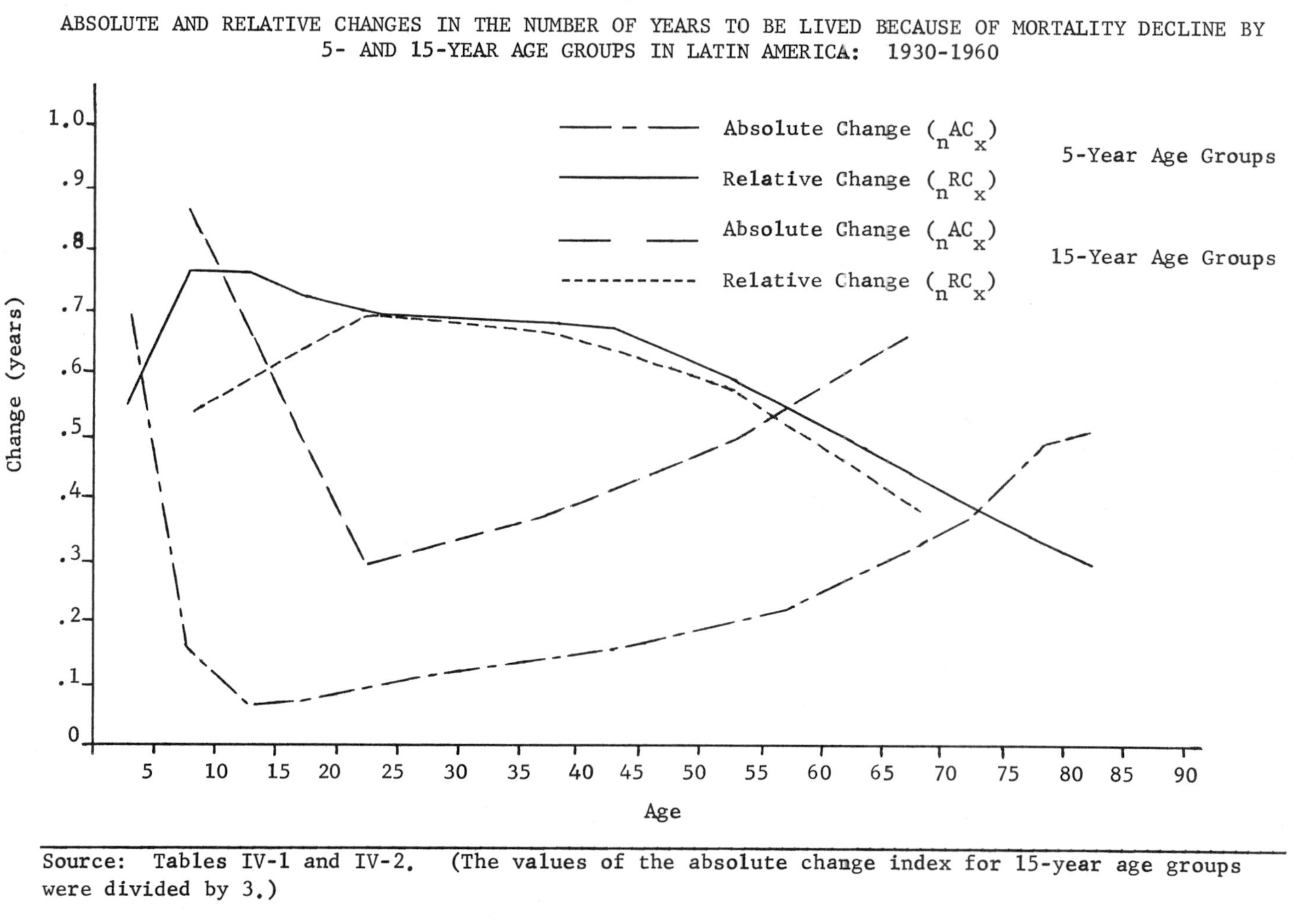

Source: Tables IV-1 and IV-2. (The values of the absolute change index for 15-year age groups were divided by 3.)

Table IV-2

TEMPORARY LIFE EXPECTANCIES FOR 5-YEAR AGE GROUPS IN LATIN AMERICA: ABSOLUTE AND RELATIVE CHANGES, BOTH SEXES, 1930's TO 1960's

(Averages for eleven Latin American countries)[a]

		Age Groups								
Index	Year(s)	0-4	5-9	10-14	15-19	20-24	25-29	30-34	35-39	40-44
$/n\ e_x$	1930	3.7290	4.7756	4.9068	4.9004	4.8621	4.8359	4.8185	4.7967	4.7671
$/n\ e_x$	1960	4.4329	4.9455	4.9776	4.9721	4.9573	4.9486	4.9428	4.9352	4.9209
$_n AC_x$	1930-60	.7039	.1699	.0708	.0717	.0952	.1127	.1243	.1385	.1538
$_n RC_x$	1930-60	.5538	.7571	.7597	.7199	.6904	.6868	.6848	.6813	.6604
		45-49	50-54	55-59	60-64	65-69	70-74	75-79	80-84	
$/n\ e_x$	1930	4.7241	4.6624	4.5750	4.4466	4.2597	3.9813	3.5891	3.1355	
$/n\ e_x$	1960	4.8969	4.8589	4.8017	4.7129	4.5735	4.3609	4.0557	3.6449	
$_n AC_x$	1930-60	.1728	.1965	.2267	.2663	.3139	.3796	.4666	.5094	
$_n RC_x$	1930-60	.5955	.5787	.5066	.4779	.4209	.3896	.3104	.2863	

[a]For listing of countries, see Table IV-1.

Source: Appendix IV, Table A-IV-2.

situation. In other words, mortality decline in young adult ages was greater than the increase of mortality because of aging during the period 1930 to 1960.[3]

The similarity of mortality decline by age in the eleven Latin American countries being discussed is not surprising considering modern communication and the interchange of medical knowledge among the countries of the world. The eleven countries have the same mortality-change pattern, and only small differences exist in the magnitude of the change.[4] Furthermore, this mortality-change pattern occurs not only in the Latin American countries, but also in countries of other regions (see Tables IV-1 and IV-3).

The similarity in the pattern of mortality change among countries with different demographic and economic characteristics requires an explanation. In Latin America, as well as in European countries, India, Japan, and Taiwan, ages under 15 received the greatest benefit in the number of years to be lived, while ages 15 to 29 received the least benefit. Nevertheless, the latter age group registered the greatest relative increase.

---

[3]For example, a Venezuelan man at age 24 in 1931 had a survivor ratio $P_x = \frac{L_{x+1}}{L_x}$ of .9869. The same person at age 29 in 1936 had a survivor ratio of .9872; at age 34 in 1941, .9879; at age 44 in 1951, .9884; and at age 54 in 1961, .9884. Venezuela was the country with the greatest mortality change in Latin America during the 30-year period starting in the 1930's. In Costa Rica, which was the Latin American country with the smallest mortality change (although the one at the lowest mortality level), the survivor ratio for a man at age 23 in 1933 was .9916; at age 33 in 1943, .9934; at age 43 in 1953, .9931; and at age 53 in 1963, .9904.

[4]Venezuela and Costa Rica are the countries with the largest and smallest changes respectively (absolute and relative changes). It should be remembered that the indices ${}_nAC_x$ and ${}_nRC_x$ measure the <u>change</u> in the number of years to be lived because of the mortality decline, but not the <u>level</u> of mortality. The change in Costa Rica occurred at the lowest mortality level of the Latin American countries. The mortality level for each country and for each age group is given by the temporary life expectancies-- $/n\ e_x^t$. (They are not compared here, but easily could be by using the information given in Appendix IV, Tables A-IV-1 and A-IV-2.)

Table IV-3

TEMPORARY LIFE EXPECTANCIES FOR 15-YEAR AGE GROUPS IN SELECTED COUNTRIES: ABSOLUTE AND RELATIVE CHANGES, BOTH SEXES, 1930's TO 1960's

Index	Year(s)	Age Groups 0-14	15-29	30-44	45-59	60-74
				EUROPE[a]		
$/n\ e_x$	1930	12.9489	14.5681	14.4022	13.8112	11.6942
$/n\ e_x$	1960	14.4714	14.9005	14.8116	14.3468	12.5343
${}_nAC_x$	1930-60	1.5225	.3324	.4094	.5356	.8401
${}_nRC_x$	1930-60	.7423	.7696	.6848	.4505	.2541
				INDIA		
$/n\ e_x$	1921-30	9.3222	13.4816	12.3712	11.1117	9.2295
$/n\ e_x$	1951-60	11.5992	14.3927	13.4294	12.0971	9.8762
${}_nAC_x$	1921-60	2.2770	.9111	1.0582	.9854	.6467
${}_nRC_x$	1921-60	.4010	.6000	.4225	.2534	.1124
				JAPAN		
$/n\ e_x$	1926-30	11.9246	14.0465	14.1338	13.2571	10.8831
$/n\ e_x$	1959-60	14.3936	14.8457	14.7370	14.2261	12.2005
${}_nAC_x$	1926-60	2.4690	.7992	.6032	.9690	1.3174
${}_nRC_x$	1926-60	.8028	.8382	.6964	.5560	.3200
				TAIWAN		
$/n\ e_x$	1936-40	11.4533	14.4127	13.8887	12.8714	10.4134
$/n\ e_x$	1959-60	13.9208	14.8284	14.6458	14.0704	11.7779
${}_nAC_x$	1936-60	2.4675	.4157	.7571	1.1990	1.3645
${}_nRC_x$	1936-60	.6957	.7082	.6813	.5633	.2975

[a]Belgium, Bulgaria, Czechoslovakia, England and Wales, France, Italy, Poland, Spain, and Sweden. The United States was also included because of its similar mortality characteristics.

Source: Appendix IV, Table A-IV-3.

Although the pattern of mortality change in developing as well as advanced countries has been the same, the causes of such similarity have been different in each case. Under the mortality circumstances of Latin American countries in the 1930's (high mortality rates in the very young ages) and with the help of "imported" medical knowledge and techniques, not only the greatest absolute change, but also the greatest relative change should have been expected to occur in ages under 15. Mortality in these ages should have declined from the high levels of the 1930's to levels as low as those registered in advanced countries.

Why did this not happen in Latin America? Why was the relative change in ages under 15 not the highest? Furthermore, why was the relative change in Europe for ages under 15 also not the greatest? The answer is different for each region. In the 1930's, in countries with previously low mortality rates, such as those in Europe, infant mortality was at such a low level that any further decline required diligent efforts, particularly to reduce deaths due to endogenous causes during the early years of life. On the other hand, in countries such as those in Latin America, where in the 1960's infant mortality could still be greatly reduced, certain factors prevented a more rapid mortality decline than the one observed. Inadequate nutrition and poor living conditions were two such factors. High fertility may also, to some extent, have limited the mortality decline in childhood years.[5] In high fertility countries, the "per-capita mother-care" received by each child is lower than in countries with low fertility.[6] It is not difficult to imagine the situation of children in poor, large families where each sibling has to share mother-care and little food. When all these factors are taken into account, the existence of high mortality rates in young children due to infectious and pulmonary respiratory diseases in some Latin American countries is not surprising.[7]

---

[5] J. Knodel and E. van del Valle, "Breast Feeding, Fertility and Infant Mortality," Population Studies, XXI, No. 2 (September 1967): 131.

[6] The average number of children born to mothers aged 45 to 49 in Venezuela was 6.3 in the 1950 census and 6.0 in the 1960 census. In Mexico it was 6.4 in the 1960 census. In Chile (the country with the lowest fertility rate among the Latin American countries considered in this study), the 1960 census shows the number of children born to mothers aged 40 to 49 to be 4.8. The proportion of mothers aged 40 to 49 who had 10 or more births was 22 percent in Mexico and 17 percent in Venezuela in 1960.

[7] Arnoldo Cabaldón, "Leading Causes of Death in Latin America," Milbank Memorial Fund Quarterly, XLIII, No. 4, Part 2 (October 1965): 242-262.

In sum, in the period from 1930 to 1960 it was relatively easier to save the life of a young adult than of a child in Latin America, as well as in Europe. In developing regions this was true because of the low standard of living combined with high fertility rates, in advanced countries because mortality at very early ages had reached levels so low that they could hardly be further reduced.

Mortality Decline by Sex

Female mortality in a population at a given moment is usually lower than male mortality, especially when the life expectancy at birth for both sexes exceeds 35 years.[8] Latin American countries are no exception to this rule. Lower female mortality has been documented in all countries in the area since the 1930's, with the exception of El Salvador and Guatemala in 1930.[9]

The difference between female and male mortality in Latin America tended to increase as mortality fell, because female mortality declined faster than male mortality. For instance, in the 1930's in the eleven countries under consideration, females had an average life expectancy at birth of 34.3 years, as against 33.3 years for males. There was no country with a difference between the life expectancies of the two sexes greater than 2.2 years. Thirty years later, however, in the 1960's, the difference on the average had increased to 3.3 years; the life expectancies for males and females were 55.2 and 58.5 years respectively. For each individual country the difference was greater than 2.7 years, ranging from 2.8 in Costa Rica to 4.5 years in Chile. (For individual countries, see Appendix IV, Table A-IV-4.) From the 1930's to the 1960's, females added an average of 24.1 years to their life expectancies at birth, whereas males added only 21.8 years. A greater increase in life expectancy for females than for males was observed for every one of the eleven Latin American countries.

How much did each sex contribute to the total population mortality decline, if the decline is measured by the life expectancies for both sexes combined? The contribution of each sex

---

[8] Among all the life tables published by the United Nations in the Demographic Yearbook (several years), the only exceptions to this pattern are Cambodia, Ceylon, India, and Pakistan.

[9] The interpolated life table of Guatemala for 1934 gives a life expectancy at birth of 26.4 for males and 26.3 for females. The life tables used for the interpolation had the following life expectancies at birth: 1921--male 26.6, female 26.1; 1940--male 30.3, female 30.5.

to the life expectancy for both sexes is not the same as the relative differences between the life expectancy increase for each sex--an increase which was 11 percent greater for females than for males. In order to determine the contribution of each sex we must consider not only the sex composition of the total population, but also the number of male and female births.

In a closed population which has had a constant masculinity[10] at birth in the past, the life expectancy for both sexes is

$$e_o^T = h.e_o^m + (1-h)\ e_o^f \qquad \text{(IV-3)}$$

where T, m, and f stand for total, male, and female, and h is the masculinity at birth.[11]

Under the above conditions, the change in the life expectancy for both sexes from year t to year t+i would be

$$^{t,t+i}e_o^T = h\ .\ \Delta^{t,t+i}\ e_o^m + (1-h)\ .\ \Delta^{t,t+i}\ e_o^f \qquad \text{(IV-4)}$$

and the percent each sex contributes to the change of the total life expectancy would be, for males:

$$MC^{t,t+i} = 100\ \frac{h\ .\ \Delta^{t,t+i}\ e_o^m}{\Delta^{t,t+i}\ e_o^T} \qquad \text{(IV-4)}$$

and for females:

$$FC^{t,t+i} = 100 - MC^{t,t+i} \qquad \text{(IV-5)}$$

The contribution of each sex to the total mortality decline depends not only on the mortality decline of each sex, but also on the sex ratio at birth. In Latin America, while females reduced mortality more rapidly than males, males were more numerous than females at birth. As a consequence, we can say that while in one respect females tended to contribute more than males to the

---

[10]A constant proportion of male births.

[11]Even when Latin American populations are not "closed" and do not have a constant masculinity at birth, they are not too far from these two conditions for the purpose of determining the contribution of each sex to the mortality change of the total population.

reduction of total mortality because female mortality decline was greater than male, in another respect males tended to contribute more than females to the total mortality decline because males were more numerous than females at birth. The two factors generally balanced one another, so that the contributions of the two sexes to the total mortality decline were never far from parity. The eleven-country average contribution of each sex was 48.7 percent for males and 51.3 percent for females from the 1930's to the 1960's. Only in Costa Rica did males contribute more than females to the total mortality decline. In Mexico, each sex contributed exactly 50 percent (see Table IV-4).

Table IV-4

CONTRIBUTION BY SEX TO THE INCREASE OF TOTAL POPULATION LIFE EXPECTANCY IN SELECTED LATIN AMERICAN COUNTRIES: 1930's TO 1960's

		Percent Contribution	
Country	Period	Male	Female
Brazil	1930-60	49.0	51.0
Chile	1930-60	46.9	53.1
Costa Rica	1933-63	50.5	49.5
El Salvador	1931-61	48.1	51.9
Guatemala	1934-64	47.0	53.0
Honduras	1931-61	49.4	50.6
Mexico	1930-60	50.0	50.0
Nicaragua	1933-63	49.1	50.9
Panama	1930-60	48.5	51.5
Paraguay	1932-62	49.1	50.9
Venezuela	1931-61	49.0	51.0

Source: Calculated from Appendix IV, Table A-IV-4, and masculinity ratios from vital statistics information published by the various countries.

Table IV-5

TEMPORARY LIFE EXPECTANCIES FOR 15-YEAR AGE GROUPS IN LATIN AMERICA: ABSOLUTE AND RELATIVE CHANGES, BY SEX, 1930's TO 1960's

(Averages for eleven Latin American countries)[a]

		Age Groups									
		Male					Female				
Index	Year(s)	0-14	15-29	30-44	45-59	60-74	0-14	15-29	30-44	45-59	60-74
$/n\ e_x$	1930	10.0405	13.9562	13.3509	12.1754	9.6791	10.2458	13.8695	13.2956	12.5695	10.2079
$/n\ e_x$	1960	12.7582	14.6513	14.4101	13.7215	11.5999	13.0682	14.6840	14.4780	14.0220	12.1970
${}_nAC_x$	1930-60	2.7177	.6951	1.0592	1.5461	1.9208	2.8224	.8145	1.1824	1.4525	1.9891
${}_nRC_x$	1930-60	.5480	.6659	.6423	.5474	.3610	.5937	.7264	.6937	.5976	.4151

[a]For listing of countries, see Table IV-1.

Source: Appendix IV-2, Table A-IV-1.

Sex Mortality Changes for Particular Ages

As in the preceding section, the indices ${}_{n}AC_{x}$ and ${}_{n}RC_{x}$ (absolute change and relative change) are used here to establish the mortality decline registered by each sex in each 15-year age group during the period 1930 to 1960. Practically all countries registered the same pattern of change. Females increased more than males the number of years to be lived in relation to the possible gain in all the countries. That is, all countries show a greater ${}_{n}RC_{x}$ index for females than for males in all the 15-year age groups. The averages of the eleven Latin American countries by age groups are:

	Age Groups				
	0-14	15-29	30-44	45-60	60-74
Male	.5480	.6659	.6423	.5474	.3610
Female	.5937	.7268	.6937	.5976	.4151
Difference: Females-Males	.0457	.0609	.0514	.0502	.0541

Source: Table IV-5. For details by country, see Appendix IV, Table A-IV-1.

The absolute change in the number of years to be lived--the ${}_{n}AC_{x}$ index--does not show as consistent a pattern as the ${}_{n}RC_{x}$ index.[12] The average for the eleven Latin American countries shows a greater absolute increase for females than for males, except in the 45-59 age group, as can be seen below.

	Age Groups				
	0-14	15-29	30-44	45-59	60-74
Male	2.72	.70	1.06	1.55	1.92
Female	2.82	.81	1.18	1.45	1.99
Difference: Females-Males	.10	.11	.12	-.10	.07

Source: Table IV-5.

[12] It must be remembered that the ${}_{n}AC_{x}$ index is affected by the temporary life expectancy which existed at the beginning of the period under study.

Table IV-6

TEMPORARY LIFE EXPECTANCIES FOR SELECTED AGE GROUPS IN LATIN AMERICA: ABSOLUTE AND RELATIVE CHANGES, BY SEX, 1930's TO 1960's

(Average for eleven Latin American countries)[a]

		Age Groups			
		Male		Female	
Index	Year(s)	15-44	20-49	15-44	20-49
$/n\ e_x$	1930	25.2920	24.4811	25.0045	24.2816
$/n\ e_x$	1960	28.3064	27.9264	28.4874	28.1897
${}_nAC_x$	1930-60	3.0144	3.4453	3.4829	3.9081
${}_nRC_x$	1930-60	.6403	.6243	.6972	.6834

[a] For listing of countries, see Table IV-1.

Source: Appendix IV, Table A-IV-5.

All countries exhibit this pattern of absolute change except Chile, Costa Rica, Mexico, Paraguay, and Venezuela, in which the male increase in ages 0-14 was slightly greater than that of females (for individual countries, see Appendix IV, Table A-IV-1).

The interesting finding in this differential sex mortality decline is that the decline within the childbearing ages was greater for females than for males, in absolute as well as relative terms. For the eleven Latin American countries, the average absolute and relative increases in the number of years to be lived were:

	Age Groups			
	Absolute Change		Relative Change in Relation to the Maximum Possible Change	
	15-44	20-49	15-44	20-49
Male	3.01	3.45	.6403	.6243
Female	3.48	3.91	.6972	.6834
Difference:				
Females-Males	.47	.46	.0569	.0591

Source: Table IV-6. (For results by country, see Appendix IV, Table A-IV-5.)

Why is the increase in the number of years to be lived during childbearing ages greater among females than among males in countries that still have high fertility? What forces operate to keep the pattern in countries of high fertility the same as that in countries of low fertility? The temporary life expectancies in childbearing ages were higher for males than for females in most of the countries in the 1930's, but the reverse was true in the 1960's. Why was there such a change if fertility was still at such a high level? A number of factors were involved.

Females have a "unique" sex cause of death which operates in connection with the reproductive process: complications in pregnancies and deliveries. In countries like those of Latin America with high fertility, the risk of a female's dying as a result of a bad pregnancy is much greater than in countries with low fertility.[13] Males, on the other hand, are not subject to an increase in the causes of death deriving from parenthood. Hence,

---

[13]This is not only because the proportion of females annually who are mothers in Latin America is higher than, for example, in Europe, but also because the mortality rate per mother is higher.

an increase in the number of years to be lived by females of childbearing ages in high-fertility areas should not be greater than that for males; nevertheless, this was the case in Latin American countries between the 1930's and the 1960's.

European countries showed exactly the same phenomenon from the 1930's to the 1960's. That is, the increase in the number of years to be lived during the female reproductive ages was smaller for males than for females, with the sex differential even greater than in Latin America (see Tables IV-5 and IV-7).

It is necessary to examine the causes of death for an explanation. Unfortunately, there is no trustworthy information concerning causes of death for Latin American countries in the 1930's; hence, our analysis is limited to the 1960's. The study of causes of death of females leads to the conclusion that in Latin America at the present time, although maternal mortality is still greater than in Europe, this cause of death does not have an important effect on the life span of females.

If the pregnancy mortality rates of Latin American countries are compared to those of European countries, a "great" difference is observed. The average annual mortality rate due to pregnancies for eight Latin American countries was .00034 for ages 15-29 and .00051 for ages 30-44 in the 1960's. For the same date and age groups the average for ten European countries and the United States was .00004 and .00006 respectively. (See Table IV-8. Rates for each country are given in Appendix IV, Tables A-IV-6 and A-IV-7.) The relative differences between the rates of both areas show that maternal mortality is higher by more than 750 percent in Latin America. What does this high percentage mean? On the average, how many years longer will a European girl live than a Latin American girl because of lower maternal mortality?[14]

In order to see what the effect is of the differential mortality in the two regions considered, it is necessary to calculate how much maternal mortality affects the number of years to be lived by the female population. Assuming that only maternal mortality affected the female population, European girls 15 years old would live an approximate average of 14 years and 363 days during the next 15 years, while Latin American girls would live 14 years and 351 days (in decimals, 14.9955 for Europe and 14.9616 for Latin America). Now it is clear how small the effect of

---

[14] This high percentage and its actual meaning demonstrate what I would call the fallacy of the relative comparison of mortality rates. This "fallacy" is one of the reasons why a comparison of mortality rates has been avoided in this study.

Table IV-7

TEMPORARY LIFE EXPECTANCIES FOR 15-YEAR AGE GROUPS IN SELECTED COUNTRIES IN EUROPE: ABSOLUTE AND RELATIVE CHANGES, BY SEX, 1930's TO 1960's[a]

		Age Groups									
		Male					Female				
Index	Year(s)	0-14	15-29	30-44	45-59	60-74	0-14	15-29	30-44	45-59	60-74
$/_n e_x$	1930	12.8101	14.5520	14.3804	13.6923	11.4237	13.0876	14.5842	14.4240	13.9301	11.9646
$/_n e_x$	1960	14.4248	14.8620	14.7692	14.1789	11.9629	14.5180	14.9390	14.8540	14.5147	13.1056
$_n AC_x$	1930-60	1.6147	.3100	.3888	.4866	.5392	1.4304	.3548	.4300	.5846	1.1410
$_n RC_x$	1930-60	.7373	.6920	.6275	.3721	.1508	.7480	.8533	.7465	.5464	.3759

[a]For listing of countries, see Table IV-3.

Source: Appendix IV, Table A-IV-3.

Table IV-8

DEATH RATES FROM SELECTED CAUSES FOR AGES 15-29 AND 30-44 IN LATIN AMERICA AND EUROPE: BY SEX, 1960's

(Per hundred thousand)

Region	Death Rates						
	Male			Female			
	Total	Accidents	Total, Minus Accidents	Total	Pregnancy	Accidents	Total, Minus Pregnancies and Accidents
				Age 15-29			
Latin America	299.51	124.49	175.02	246.88	34.21	20.54	192.13
Europe	134.93	81.00	53.93	63.03	3.96	16.42	42.65
				Age 30-44			
Latin America	571.87	178.03	393.85	472.96	50.57	20.61	401.78
Europe	267.96	85.41	182.55	162.07	5.75	18.95	137.37

Source: Appendix IV, Tables A-IV-6 and A-IV-7.

differential maternal mortality is, or rather how small the difference between the actual case and the hypothetical case of no maternal deaths at all--almost 15 years would be lived in both cases. If instead of ages 15 to 29 the age group 30 to 44 is analyzed, there is again not much difference. Under the same circumstances, European females would live 14.9935 years and Latin American females 14.9432 years. The life span of females is affected very little by maternal mortality. In other words, differential fertility in the two populations has virtually no effect on mortality during the reproductive ages, but does affect the offspring population generated by fertility, as was noted above (see footnote 5). The cause of death "unique" to females has practically no effect on their life span.

Do any sex-specific death factors operate within the male population? One cause of death, though not "exclusively" acting on males, almost by itself produces the difference in mortality rates between the sexes--namely, accidents. Male accidents are so numerous that startling results are obtained if mortality rates for both sexes for the age group 15 to 29 are compared. For eight Latin American countries having information, the average male accident mortality rate represents more than one-half of the total female mortality rate. For the European countries, the average male accident rates are higher than the total female mortality rate. (See Table IV-8. In the same table, accident mortality rates for males can be compared with accident-plus-pregnancy mortality rates for females and, in addition, rates for all the remaining [unspecified] causes of death in each sex.)

The levels of accident mortality rates in Europe and Latin America differ less than the death rates from "other causes." In other words, the differential of male accident mortality between Europe and Latin America is not as great as for the other causes of death.[15] The male European accident rate in the age group 15 to 29 has not declined as rapidly as the other causes of death. The male accident rate in Europe has remained high in comparison with the total female mortality rate. Accidents are one of the most difficult causes of death to reduce. This circumstance, together with the fact that males are the principal accident victims, explains why in Latin America, as well as in Europe, the increase in the number of years to be lived from age 15 to 29 was less for males than for females. It is also clear now why the relative increase of years to be lived for European males from age 15 to 29 changed so little--less than that for males under

---

[15] An average of 43 per hundred thousand more males die in Latin America than in Europe because of accidents, while 121 per hundred thousand more males die in Latin America than in Europe because of "other" causes of death.

age 15, and almost equal to the increase in Latin America for ages 15-29. For females, the relative increase for ages 15-29 was much greater in Europe than in Latin America (Tables IV-5 and IV-7).

For males and females aged 30 to 44 the same cause-of-death phenomenon as in the preceding age group is repeated, although the rapid increase in "other causes" of death makes accidents relatively less important. (Details for each country are in Appendix IV, Table A-IV-7.)

Summary

A noticeable consequence of the rapid mortality decline in Latin America during the period 1930 to 1960 was the increase in the number of life-years in childhood ages. Young adult ages benefitted the least in absolute terms. However, young adults, principally females, registered the largest increase relative to the maximum possible increase in the number of years to be lived. Despite the high fertility rate in Latin America, maternal mortality has had no significant effect on the female life span, while accidents have prevented a rapid mortality decline among young males. Consequently, in the childbearing (young adult) ages during the 1930-1960 period, females increased their life span more than males.

Appendix IV

Interpolation of the Life Tables

The analysis of mortality in Latin America is made for the 30-year period with the most rapid mortality decline, which, in all the selected countries, begins in the 1930's and ends in the 1960's (at least until the 1970 data are available).

A life table for the 1960's and another for 30 or more years earlier are required if a country is to be included in the analysis. This limits the number of countries to be analyzed to eleven. Bolivia, Haiti, and Colombia were eliminated because they do not have a life table for the 1960's; the Dominican Republic, Ecuador, and Peru because they do not have one for the 1930's or even before. Only Brazil, Chile, Costa Rica, El Salvador, Guatemala, Honduras, Mexico, Nicaragua, Panama, Paraguay, and Venezuela remain. The interval between the two life tables to be analyzed must of necessity be 30 years, in order to equalize the period of analysis. Among the eleven countries, Chile, Mexico, and Panama have life tables for both 1960 and 1930. For the remaining countries, the ${}_5L_x$ values were interpolated by using a polynomial function. The degree of the polynomial depended on the number of pivotal points, which were as many as the number of life tables constructed for each country. The degree of the polynomial for each country was second degree for El Salvador; third degree for Honduras, Nicaragua, and Paraguay; fourth degree for Guatemala; and fifth degree for Brazil and Costa Rica. Venezuela was a special case where an exponential interpolation between 1926 and 1936 was made. The dates of interpolation for each case and the nearest life table years between which the interpolation fell were as follows:

Country	Year of Interpolation	Nearest Life Table Years Between Which the Interpolation Fell
Brazil	1930	1920-1940
Costa Rica	1933	1927-1950
El Salvador	1931	1930-1950
Guatemala	1934	1921-1940
Honduras	1931	1930-1940
Nicaragua	1930	1920-1940
Paraguay	1932	1899-1950
Venezuela	1931	1926-1936

In all cases, the function used for each interpolated value of $_5L_x$ did not have its maximum or minimum within the interval of interpolation; in other words, the functions were monotonously increasing. The life expectancies at birth of the interpolated values, and those life expectancies for the adjacent pivotal values can be seen in the following table.

Country	Life Expectancies (years)		
	Early Life Table to the Interpolated Date	Interpolated Values	Life Table After the Interpolated Date
Brazil	32.0	33.6	36.7
Costa Rica	40.0	43.5	55.5
El Salvador	28.7	29.6	47.2
Guatemala	25.8	26.3	30.4
Honduras	34.0	34.3	37.5
Nicaragua	24.3	31.3	34.5
Paraguay	26.1	35.6	45.8
Venezuela	32.2	33.0	33.9

Indices Used in the Analysis of Mortality Decline

From among the indices used in the measurement of mortality, the most appropriate for the purposes of this study were selected. The study concerns the effect of mortality decline on the age structure of the population--in other words, the increase of certain age groups faster than others. If the population under age x has grown faster than that over age x, the structure of the population changes with the proportion of people in ages under x greater than before. For example, if the increase in the number of years to be lived up to age 35 by those alive at birth has been greater than the increase in the number of years to be lived up to age 70 by those persons alive at age 35, the proportion of persons in ages under 35 will increase. (For a mathematical explanation of the effect of mortality on the age structure, see Chapter V.)

Changes in the age structure due to changes in mortality are more understandable if the decline of mortality is measured in terms of the number of years to be lived rather than the number of deaths--more specifically, by indices which consider the number of years lived during ages x to x+n by those alive at age x. The life tables provide good indices to analyze mortality change by age--specifically, the L_x function.

APPENDIX IV

The L_x function can represent a stationary population, the survivors from birth within age x and x+1, or the average number of years to be lived between age x and x+1 by the life table births l_o (the three concepts under the hypothetical mortality-fertility conditions of the life table). When referring to the number of years which, on the average, will be lived by the births (the radix of the life table, l_o) within the ages x and x+1, the L_x term can be divided by those alive at exact age x, that is l_x. Hence,

$$\frac{L_x}{l_x} \qquad \text{(A-IV-1)}$$

gives the number of years to be lived during age x and x+1 by those alive at age x. If instead of one age, a group of n ages is considered, the result is a temporary n life expectancy[1] at age x, which in symbols is

$$/n\; e_x = \frac{\sum_{i=0}^{n-1} L_{x+i}}{l_x} = \frac{T_x - T_{x+n}}{l_x} \qquad \text{(A-IV-2)}$$

The male life table for Panama for 1930 provides an illustrative numerical example.[2] The L_x and l_x functions for this table are:

Age	L_x	l_x	$\frac{L_x}{l_o}$	$\frac{L_x}{l_x}$
	(1)	(2)	(3)	(4)
15	63512	63658	.6351	.9977
20	61242	61483	.6124	.9961
25	58285	58592	.5828	.9948
30	55091	55409	.5509	.9943
35	51725	52060	.5172	.9934
40	48002	48374	.4800	.9923
45	43741	44170	.4374	.9903

[1] Galé, Matemáticas Financieras (Segunda Parte).

[2] Arriaga, New Life Tables. The life table for Panama gives the L_x function for 5-year age groups. They were broken down by using Beers' coefficients (H.S. Beers, "Six-Term Formulas for Routine Actuarial Interpolation," Records of the American Institute of Actuaries, XXXIV [June 1945]: 60).

The tabulation indicates that, on the average, the newborn male baby in Panama in 1930 would have lived only .6351 years between age 15 and 16 (column 3) under the mortality conditions of the time. Similarly, those alive at exact age 15 would have lived on the average .9977 years during ages 15 and 16 (column 4). If instead of single ages, the ${}_5L_x$ are considered--that is, 5-year age groups--the values are:

Age Group	${}_5L_x$	$\frac{{}_5L_x}{l_o}$	$\frac{{}_5L_x}{l_x}$ *
15-19	313541	3.1354	4.9254
20-24	300493	3.0049	4.8874
25-29	285028	2.8503	4.8646
30-34	268815	2.6882	4.8515
35-39	251361	2.5136	4.8283
40-44	231745	2.3174	4.7907
45-49	209220	2.0922	4.7367

*Same l_x as before.

According to this table, those newborn in 1930 would have lived on the average only 3.1354 years between age 15 and 20, or those who were alive at exact age 15 would have lived on the average 4.9254 years between ages 15 and 20 under constant 1930 mortality. For wider intervals of age--for instance, 15 years--the life table gives the following figures:

Age Group	ΣL_x	$\frac{\Sigma L_x}{l_o}$	$/15\ e_x = \frac{\Sigma L_x}{l_x}$
15-29	959062	9.5906	14.1233
30-44	751921	7.5192	13.5704

The interpretation is the same as before. The change during a period of time in the number of years to be lived by a population within certain ages is obtained by comparing two temporary life expectancies.[3] For instance, the temporary life expectancies

[3] The comparison can be made not only for the same population, but also for different countries or regions and the two sexes.

for males aged 15-29 and 30-44 in Panama in the years 1930 and 1960 were:

	$/15\ e_x$		Difference
	1930	1960	(2) - (1)
Age Group	(1)	(2)	(3)
15-29	14.1233	14.7253	.6020
30-44	13.5704	14.5720	1.0016

Column (3) gives the increase in the number of years to be lived between ages 15 and 30 for those alive at exact age 15, or between ages 30 and 45 for those alive at exact age 30, due to the change of mortality conditions from the 1930's to 1960. In symbols, the change of the two life expectancies can be indicated as

$$_nAC_x^{t,t+i} = /n\ e_x^{t+i} - /n\ e_x^{t} \qquad \text{(A-IV-3)}$$

where t and t+i refer to the years in which the life tables were constructed (1930 and 1960 in this case). The absolute change of temporary life expectancy--$_nAC_x^{t,t+i}$--depends on the possible change that can occur. In the given case, for ages 15-29 the increase of the temporary life expectancy cannot be more than .8767 years. In other words, the temporary life expectancy--$/ne_x$--cannot have values over n (here 15), which would only be reached if no person died during the age interval. Therefore, for some cases, it would be useful to calculate a relative measurement of the mortality change, the registered change measured in relation to the possible or maximum change--that is, n minus the temporary life expectancy at the earlier date (in symbols, $n - /n\ e_x^t$). The relative change would be

$$_nRC_x^{t,t+i} = \frac{_nAC_x^{t,t+i}}{n - /n\ e_x^t} \qquad \text{(A-IV-4)}$$

Using the figures from Panama, the absolute change was greater for ages 30-44 than for ages 15-29, but if the relative change is calculated, the values are:

Age Group	$_{15}AC_x^{30,60}$	$_{15}RC_x^{30,60}$
15-29	.6020	.6376
30-44	1.0016	.6212

Both indices AC and RC are used in the text.

In calculating these indices, it is also possible to consider more than one age. For this study, it would be useful to have the index for two ages--or lives--in order to measure the effect of the mortality decline on the life spans of a married couple (or consensual union) considered as a unit. If, for instance, y is the age of the man and x the age of the woman, the temporary life expectancy for two lives is defined as

$$/n\ e_{x:y} = \overset{o}{e}_{x:y} - {}_nP_{x:y} \cdot \overset{o}{e}_{x+n:y+n} \qquad \text{(A-IV-5)}$$

where

$$ {}_nP_{x:y} = \frac{l_{x+n} \cdot l_{y+n}}{l_x \cdot l_y} \qquad \text{(A-IV-6)}$$

Formula A-IV-5 can be rewritten as:

$$/n\ e_{x:y} = \frac{\sum_{j=o}^{n-1} L_{x+j:y+j}}{l_{x:y}} \qquad \text{(A-IV-7)}$$

where

$$L_{x:y} = L_x \cdot L_y \qquad \text{(A-IV-8)}$$

and

$$l_{x:y} = l_x \cdot l_y \qquad \text{(A-IV-9)}$$

for the cases when the life table functions are for single ages. If, as usual, we have 5-year age groups (abridged life tables) the ${}_5L_{x:y}$ would keep its structure:

$${}_5L_{x:y} = {}_5L_x \cdot {}_5L_y \qquad \text{(A-IV-10)}$$

but the temporary life expectancy must be calculated as

$$/n\ e_{x:y} = \frac{\sum_{j=o}^{k-1} {}_5L_{x+5j:y+5j}}{5\ .\ l_{x:y}} \qquad \text{(A-IV-11)}$$

where $k = \frac{n}{5}$. As previously, the two indices for two persons are:

$${}_nAC^{t,t+i}_{x:y} = /n\ e^{t+i}_{x:y} - /n\ e^{t}_{x:y} \qquad \text{(A-IV-12)}$$

and

$${}_nRC^{t,t+i}_{x:y} = \frac{{}_nAC^{t,t+i}_{x:y}}{n - /n\ e^{t}_{x:y}} \qquad \text{(A-IV-13)}$$

The meaning of these two indices is the same as when they are applied to only one life; in the present case, two persons are considered as a unit. The unit is "alive" only while both persons remain alive.

Table A-IV-1

TEMPORARY LIFE EXPECTANCIES FOR 15-YEAR AGE GROUPS IN ELEVEN SELECTED LATIN AMERICAN COUNTRIES: ABSOLUTE AND RELATIVE CHANGES, BY SEX, 1930's TO 1960's

		Age Groups									
		Male					Female				
Index	Year	0-14	15-29	30-44	45-59	60-74	0-14	15-29	30-44	45-59	60-74
						BRAZIL					
$/n\ e_x$	1930	10.0874	13.8927	13.3358	12.1893	9.7236	10.3232	13.8069	13.2698	12.5815	10.2686
$/n\ e_x$	1960	12.6623	14.5999	14.4017	13.7365	11.5549	12.9427	14.6171	14.4418	14.0037	12.1415
${}_nAC_x$	1930-60	2.5749	.7073	1.0659	1.5473	1.8312	2.6194	.8102	1.1720	1.4222	1.8728
${}_nRC_x$	1930-60	.5241	.6387	.6405	.5505	.3471	.5601	.6791	.6774	.5881	.3958
						CHILE					
$/n\ e_x$	1930	10.2115	14.0258	13.4778	12.3293	9.8051	10.4624	13.9398	13.4198	12.7373	10.3697
$/n\ e_x$	1960	12.8047	14.7001	14.3129	13.4573	11.2022	12.9250	14.7771	14.5237	13.9996	12.1516
${}_nAC_x$	1930-60	2.5932	.6743	.8351	1.1280	1.3970	2.4627	.8373	1.1038	1.2623	1.7820
${}_nRC_x$	1930-60	.5415	.6922	.5486	.4223	.2689	.5427	.7898	.6986	.5579	.3848
						COSTA RICA					
$/n\ e_x$	1933	11.3238	14.2711	13.9223	13.0365	10.6403	11.5945	14.2407	13.9229	13.3880	11.2410
$/n\ e_x$	1963	13.3623	14.8318	14.6608	14.1780	12.2448	13.5810	14.8770	14.7170	14.2802	12.5820

${}_{n}AC_{x}$	1933-63	2.0385	.5606	.7385	1.1415	1.6046	1.9866	.6363	.7941	.8922	1.3410
${}_{n}RC_{x}$	1933-63	.5545	.7692	.6853	.5813	.3680	.5833	.8380	.7373	.5535	.3567

EL SALVADOR

$/n\ e_{x}$	1931	9.5237	13.7686	13.0998	11.8135	9.3333	9.4789	13.7192	12.9851	12.1439	9.7457
$/n\ e_{x}$	1961	12.6846	14.6256	14.4271	13.7601	11.5732	12.9655	14.6429	14.4672	14.0281	12.1613
${}_{n}AC_{x}$	1931-61	3.1609	.8570	1.3273	1.9466	2.2399	3.4866	.9237	1.4821	1.8842	2.4156
${}_{n}RC_{x}$	1931-61	.5772	.6959	.6985	.6109	.3953	.6315	.7212	.7355	.6597	.4597

GUATEMALA

$/n\ e_{x}$	1934	8.8998	13.7442	12.8490	11.1881	8.4476	9.0724	13.4889	12.6158	11.6029	8.9900
$/n\ e_{x}$	1964	12.1039	14.4881	14.2322	13.4811	11.1964	12.6082	14.4870	14.2903	13.8354	11.9134
${}_{n}AC_{x}$	1934-64	3.2041	.7438	1.3831	2.2930	2.7488	3.5358	.9981	1.6745	2.2325	2.9234
${}_{n}RC_{x}$	1934-64	.5252	.5923	.6430	.6015	.4195	.5965	.6605	.7023	.6572	.4864

HONDURAS

$/n\ e_{x}$	1931	10.1668	13.9325	13.3951	12.2647	9.7740	10.4108	13.8453	13.3335	12.6639	10.3288
$/n\ e_{x}$	1961	12.4377	14.6051	14.3777	13.6661	11.4235	12.7200	14.6159	14.4172	13.9565	12.0112
${}_{n}AC_{x}$	1931-61	2.2708	.6726	.9827	1.4013	1.6495	2.3092	.7706	1.0836	1.2925	1.6824
${}_{n}RC_{x}$	1931-61	.4698	.6301	.6123	.5123	.3156	.5032	.6674	.6503	.5533	.3602

Table A-IV-1 (continued)

		Age Groups									
		Male					Female				
Index	Year	0-14	15-29	30-44	45-59	60-74	0-14	15-29	30-44	45-59	60-74
						MEXICO					
$/n\ e_x$	1930	10.0531	13.9842	13.1989	12.2474	10.0706	10.1818	14.0489	13.3891	12.6700	10.4464
$/n\ e_x$	1960	13.0389	14.6443	14.2744	13.6029	12.0124	13.1616	14.7228	14.4558	13.9710	12.3288
${}_nAC_x$	1930-60	2.9858	.6601	1.0755	1.3556	1.9418	2.9797	.6740	1.0666	1.3010	1.8824
${}_nRC_x$	1930-60	.6036	.6499	.5971	.4925	.3939	.6184	.7086	.6621	.5584	.4134
						NICARAGUA					
$/n\ e_x$	1933	9.6847	13.8088	13.1807	11.9697	9.5042	9.9091	13.7371	13.1307	12.3743	10.0686
$/n\ e_x$	1963	12.1708	14.5683	14.3108	13.5539	11.2525	12.4578	14.5712	14.3436	13.8589	11.8401
${}_nAC_x$	1933-63	2.4861	.7595	1.1301	1.5842	1.7483	2.5486	.8341	1.2129	1.4846	1.7715
${}_nRC_x$	1933-63	.4677	.6376	.6212	.5228	.3181	.5006	.6604	.6489	.5654	.3592
						PANAMA					
$/n\ e_x$	1930	10.2817	14.1233	13.5704	12.4111	9.8639	10.4957	13.9848	13.4625	12.7769	10.3991
$/n\ e_x$	1960	13.3412	14.7253	14.5720	13.9631	11.8795	13.5729	14.7630	14.6244	14.2187	12.4959

${}_nAC_x$	1930-60	3.0595	.6020	1.0016	1.5519	2.0156	3.0772	.7782	1.1619	1.4418	2.0968
${}_nRC_x$	1930-60	.6484	.6866	.7006	.5995	.3924	.6832	.7665	.7557	.6486	.4557
						PARAGUAY					
$/n\ e_x$	1932	10.2524	14.0776	13.5220	12.3574	9.6944	10.5570	13.9511	13.4724	12.7787	10.2416
$/n\ e_x$	1962	12.6733	14.6125	14.4143	13.7481	11.5640	12.9520	14.6277	14.4522	14.0138	12.1496
${}_nAC_x$	1932-62	2.4209	.5349	.8923	1.3907	1.8696	2.3950	.6766	.9798	1.2351	1.9080
${}_nRC_x$	1932-62	.5099	.5799	.6037	.5263	.3524	.5390	.6450	.6414	.5560	.4010
						VENEZUELA					
$/n\ e_x$	1931	9.9612	13.8898	13.3086	12.1226	9.6136	10.2176	13.8021	13.2496	12.5471	10.1879
$/n\ e_x$	1961	13.7182	14.7638	14.5279	13.7897	11.6959	13.8634	14.8225	14.6104	14.0766	12.2919
${}_nAC_x$	1931-61	3.7570	.8740	1.2192	1.6671	2.0823	3.6458	1.0205	1.3608	1.5295	2.1040
${}_nRC_x$	1931-61	.7456	.7873	.7208	.5794	.3866	.7623	.8519	.7774	.6235	.4372

Source: Calculated from Eduardo Arriaga, New Life Tables for Latin American Populations in the Nineteenth and Twentieth Centuries (Berkeley: International Population and Urban Research, Institute of International Studies, University of California, 1968). [Population Monograph Series No. 3]

Table A-IV-2

TEMPORARY LIFE EXPECTANCIES FOR 5-YEAR AGE GROUPS IN SELECTED LATIN AMERICAN COUNTRIES: ABSOLUTE AND RELATIVE CHANGES, BY SEX, 1930's TO 1960's

Index	Year(s)	0-4	5-9	10-14	15-19	20-24	25-29	30-34	35-39	40-44
					BRAZIL Male					
$/5\ e_x$	1930	3.7014	4.7699	4.9029	4.8982	4.8599	4.8366	4.8228	4.7992	4.7607
$/5\ e_x$	1960	4.3541	4.9280	4.9729	4.9671	4.9488	4.9404	4.9384	4.9311	4.9153
$_5AC_x$	1930-60	.6526	.1581	.0700	.0689	.0889	.1038	.1156	.1320	.1546
$_5RC_x$	1930-60	.5026	.6870	.7213	.6770	.6344	.6350	.6524	.6570	.6460
					Female					
$/5\ e_x$	1930	3.7904	4.7679	4.8958	4.8883	4.8499	4.8232	4.8073	4.7916	4.7738
$/5\ e_x$	1960	4.4436	4.9313	4.9722	4.9671	4.9520	4.9437	4.9406	4.9360	4.9272
$_5AC_x$	1930-60	.6532	.1633	.0764	.0787	.1021	.1206	.1333	.1444	.1534
$_5RC_x$	1930-60	.5400	.7038	.7335	.7052	.6802	.6818	.6916	.6927	.6783

Index	Year(s)	45-49	50-54	55-59	60-64	65-69	70-74	75-79	80-84
					Male				
$/5\ e_x$	1930	4.7062	4.6365	4.5422	4.4115	4.2253	3.9492	3.5715	3.1076
$/5\ e_x$	1960	4.8876	4.8433	4.7776	4.6786	4.5278	4.3018	3.9784	3.5305
$_5AC_x$	1930-60	.1814	.2068	.2354	.2671	.3025	.3525	.4069	.4229
$_5RC_x$	1930-60	.6173	.5689	.5142	.4539	.3905	.3355	.2848	.2235
					Female				
$/5\ e_x$	1930	4.7453	4.6956	4.6203	4.5009	4.3189	4.0526	3.6729	3.1937
$/5\ e_x$	1960	4.9094	4.8787	4.8310	4.7509	4.6171	4.4040	4.0865	3.6482
$_5AC_x$	1930-60	.1641	.1831	.2108	.2500	.2982	.3514	.4136	.4545
$_5RC_x$	1930-60	.6442	.6015	.5551	.5009	.4378	.3709	.3117	.2516

Table A-IV-2 (continued)

Index	Year(s)	0-4	5-9	10-14	15-19	20-24	25-29	30-34	35-39	40-44
					CHILE					
					Male					
$/5\ e_x$	1930	3.7211	4.7877	4.9188	4.9138	4.8759	4.8531	4.8400	4.8169	4.7793
$/5\ e_x$	1960	4.3586	4.9783	4.9831	4.9743	4.9598	4.9465	4.9329	4.9153	4.8891
$_5AC_x$	1930-60	.6375	.1906	.0644	.0605	.0839	.0934	.0929	.0983	.1098
$_5RC_x$	1930-60	.4985	.8977	.7922	.7019	.6763	.6358	.5807	.5371	.4975
					Female					
$/5\ e_x$	1930	3.8147	4.7858	4.9114	4.9037	4.8661	4.8403	4.8253	4.8106	4.7936
$/5\ e_x$	1960	4.3987	4.9813	4.9867	4.9805	4.9706	4.9616	4.9524	4.9422	4.9288
$_5AC_x$	1930-60	.5840	.1955	.0753	.0767	.1045	.1212	.1271	.1316	.1352
$_5RC_x$	1930-60	.4927	.9127	.8496	.7969	.7807	.7593	.7276	.6948	.6549

Index	Year(s)	45-49	50-54	55-59	60-64	65-69	70-74	75-79	80-84
					Male				
$/5\ e_x$	1930	4.7255	4.6557	4.5604	4.4284	4.2388	3.9558	3.5657	3.0773
$/5\ e_x$	1960	4.8525	4.7995	4.7239	4.6176	4.4593	4.2294	3.9240	3.5583
$_5AC_x$	1930-60	.1269	.1438	.1635	.1892	.2204	.2736	.3583	.4810
$_5RC_x$	1930-60	.4625	.4176	.3720	.3309	.2896	.2620	.2498	.2502
					Female				
$/5\ e_x$	1930	4.7656	4.7163	4.6408	4.5201	4.3347	4.0618	3.6689	3.1654
$/5\ e_x$	1960	4.9073	4.8717	4.8180	4.7361	4.6009	4.3910	4.0946	3.7120
$_5AC_x$	1930-60	.1417	.1554	.1771	.2160	.2662	.3291	.4257	.5466
$_5RC_x$	1930-60	.6046	.5478	.4932	.4500	.4001	.3508	.3198	.2979

Table A-IV-2 (continued)

Index	Year(s)	0-4	5-9	10-14	15-19	20-24	25-29	30-34	35-39	40-44
					COSTA RICA					
					Male					
$/5\ e_x$	1933	4.0098	4.8577	4.9436	4.9368	4.9072	4.8919	4.8865	4.8735	4.8490
$/5\ e_x$	1963	4.5339	4.9788	4.9879	4.9848	4.9780	4.9729	4.9672	4.9587	4.9455
$_5AC_x$	1933-63	.5241	.1211	.0443	.0480	.0709	.0810	.0807	.0852	.0965
$_5RC_x$	1933-63	.5293	.8509	.7855	.7595	.7635	.7489	.7109	.6737	.6392
					Female					
$/5\ e_x$	1933	4.1023	4.8593	4.9401	4.9322	4.9046	4.8881	4.8813	4.8744	4.8634
$/5\ e_x$	1963	4.6016	4.9816	4.9906	4.9891	4.9832	4.9813	4.9736	4.9649	4.9524
$_5AC_x$	1933-63	.4993	.1223	.0505	.0570	.0786	.0933	.0923	.0905	.0890
$_5RC_x$	1933-63	.5562	.8693	.8436	.8400	.8238	.8330	.7773	.7203	.6516

Index	Year(s)	45-49	50-54	55-59	60-64	65-69	70-74	75-79	80-84
					Male				
$/5\ e_x$	1933	4.8096	4.7525	4.6713	4.5544	4.3825	4.1277	3.7763	3.3221
$/5\ e_x$	1963	4.9259	4.8948	4.8436	4.7554	4.6073	4.3830	4.0621	3.6459
$_5AC_x$	1933-63	.1163	.1422	.1723	.2010	.2249	.2552	.2859	.3238
$_5RC_x$	1933-63	.6109	.5748	.5242	.4510	.3641	.2926	.2336	.1930
					Female				
$/5\ e_x$	1933	4.8413	4.8017	4.7405	4.6396	4.4794	4.2352	3.8791	3.4124
$/5\ e_x$	1963	4.9351	4.9084	4.8639	4.7874	4.6601	4.4661	4.1841	3.8061
$_5AC_x$	1933-63	.0938	.1067	.1234	.1478	.1808	.2310	.3050	.3937
$_5RC_x$	1933-63	.5912	.5381	.4756	.4101	.3472	.3020	.2721	.2480

Table A-IV-2 (continued)

Index	Year(s)	0-4	5-9	10-14	15-19	20-24	25-29	30-34	35-39	40-44
		Age Groups								
					EL SALVADOR					
					Male					
$/5\ e_x$	1931	3.5562	4.7263	4.8879	4.8855	4.8442	4.8171	4.7980	4.7676	4.7213
$/5\ e_x$	1961	4.3566	4.9310	4.9759	4.9700	4.9517	4.9432	4.9414	4.9340	4.9182
$_5AC_x$	1931-61	.8004	.2047	.0881	.0845	.1075	.1252	.1434	.1665	.1969
$_5RC_x$	1931-61	.5544	.7478	.7852	.7382	.6898	.6897	.7098	.7161	.7065
					Female					
$/5\ e_x$	1931	3.5644	4.7089	4.8869	4.8824	4.8376	4.8036	4.7783	4.7523	4.7260
$/5\ e_x$	1961	4.4462	4.9342	4.9752	4.9700	4.9549	4.9467	4.9435	4.9389	4.9301
$_5AC_x$	1931-61	.8819	.2254	.0883	.0876	.1174	.1431	.1652	.1866	.2042
$_5RC_x$	1931-61	.6143	.7741	.7804	.7451	.7226	.7285	.7451	.7532	.7450

Index	Year(s)	45-49	50-54	55-59	60-64	65-69	70-74	75-79	80-84
					Male				
$/5\ e_x$	1931	4.6584	4.5819	4.4820	4.3463	4.1544	3.8649	3.4623	2.9596
$/5\ e_x$	1961	4.8904	4.8461	4.7804	4.6813	4.5305	4.3043	3.9808	3.5324
$_5AC_x$	1931-61	.2320	.2642	.2984	.3350	.3761	.4394	.5185	.5728
$_5RC_x$	1931-61	.6792	.6319	.5760	.5125	.4448	.3871	.3372	.2807
					Female				
$/5\ e_x$	1931	4.6914	4.6345	4.5506	4.4215	4.2259	3.9406	3.5259	2.9946
$/5\ e_x$	1961	4.9123	4.8816	4.8339	4.7537	4.6198	4.4067	4.0890	3.6503
$_5AC_x$	1931-61	.2209	.2472	.2833	.3323	.3939	.4661	.5630	.6557
$_5RC_x$	1931-61	.7158	.6761	.6304	.5743	.5089	.4399	.3820	.3270

Table A-IV-2 (continued)

Index	Year(s)	Age Groups 0-4	5-9	10-14	15-19	20-24	25-29	30-34	35-39	40-44
					GUATEMALA					
					Male					
$/5\ e_x$	1934	3.3818	4.6827	4.8866	4.8871	4.8397	4.8053	4.7759	4.7320	4.6671
$/5\ e_x$	1964	4.2061	4.9032	4.9642	4.9576	4.9343	4.9231	4.9201	4.9110	4.8922
$_5AC_x$	1934-64	.8242	.2205	.0776	.0706	.0946	.1178	.1442	.1790	.2251
$_5RC_x$	1934-64	.5094	.6949	.6842	.6249	.5904	.6051	.6436	.6679	.6762
					Female					
$/5\ e_x$	1934	3.4705	4.6650	4.8619	4.8576	4.8082	4.7684	4.7358	4.7019	4.6675
$/5\ e_x$	1964	4.3655	4.9108	4.9595	4.9537	4.9363	4.9267	4.9232	4.9183	4.9092
$_5AC_x$	1934-64	.8951	.2458	.0976	.0961	.1281	.1583	.1874	.2165	.2417
$_5RC_x$	1934-64	.5852	.7337	.7064	.6752	.6679	.6836	.7093	.7261	.7270

Index	Year(s)	45-49	50-54	55-59	60-64	65-69	70-74	75-79	80-84
					Male				
$/5\ e_x$	1934	4.5824	4.4841	4.3604	4.1971	3.9742	3.6338	3.1453	2.5257
$/5\ e_x$	1964	4.8596	4.8107	4.7393	4.6325	4.4719	4.2326	3.8939	3.4333
$_5AC_x$	1934-64	.2773	.3266	.3789	.4354	.4977	.5987	.7486	.9076
$_5RC_x$	1934-64	.6639	.6331	.5924	.5423	.4852	.4383	.4036	.3668
					Female				
$/5\ e_x$	1934	4.6242	4.5553	4.4549	4.3032	4.0783	3.7539	3.2784	2.6644
$/5\ e_x$	1964	4.8906	4.8582	4.8077	4.7232	4.5835	4.3631	4.0368	3.5920
$_5AC_x$	1934-64	.2663	.3029	.3528	.4200	.5053	.6092	.7584	.9276
$_5RC_x$	1934-64	.7088	.6812	.6472	.6028	.5482	.4889	.4405	.3972

Table A-IV-2 (continued)

Index	Year(s)	0-4	5-9	10-14	15-19	20-24	25-29	30-34	35-39	40-44
		Age Groups								
					HONDURAS					
					Male					
$/5\ e_x$	1931	3.7192	4.7776	4.9073	4.9025	4.8648	4.8423	4.8295	4.8068	4.7697
$/5\ e_x$	1961	4.2869	4.9229	4.9755	4.9693	4.9486	4.9388	4.9363	4.9282	4.9110
$_5AC_x$	1931-61	.5677	.1453	.0682	.0668	.0838	.0965	.1067	.1214	.1413
$_5RC_x$	1931-61	.4432	.6535	.7360	.6851	.6201	.6119	.6261	.6283	.6137
					Female					
$/5\ e_x$	1931	3.8111	4.7754	4.8999	4.8923	4.8548	4.8291	4.8144	4.7999	4.7833
$/5\ e_x$	1961	4.3786	4.9256	4.9743	4.9686	4.9511	4.9414	4.9380	4.9330	4.9239
$_5AC_x$	1931-61	.5675	.1501	.0743	.0763	.0963	.1123	.1236	.1331	.1406
$_5RC_x$	1931-61	.4773	.6686	.7428	.7083	.6630	.6573	.6659	.6651	.6487

Index	Year(s)	45-49	50-54	55-59	60-64	65-69	70-74	75-79	80-84
					Male				
$/5\ e_x$	1931	4.7162	4.6470	4.5529	4.4217	4.2338	3.9536	3.5679	3.0859
$/5\ e_x$	1961	4.8805	4.8340	4.7660	4.6630	4.5072	4.2744	3.9434	3.4886
$_5AC_x$	1931-61	.1644	.1870	.2131	.2412	.2734	.3208	.3755	.4027
$_5RC_x$	1931-61	.5791	.5298	.4766	.4172	.3568	.3066	.2622	.2104
					Female				
$/5\ e_x$	1931	4.7557	4.7068	4.6320	4.5121	4.3286	4.0583	3.6697	3.1729
$/5\ e_x$	1961	4.9052	4.8727	4.8220	4.7373	4.5972	4.3762	4.0490	3.6022
$_5AC_x$	1931-61	.1495	.1660	.1900	.2252	.2687	.3173	.3794	.4293
$_5RC_x$	1931-61	.6120	.5659	.5164	.4616	.4001	.3375	.2852	.2350

Table A-IV-2 (continued)

Index	Year(s)	Age Groups								
		0-4	5-9	10-14	15-19	20-24	25-29	30-34	35-39	40-44
					MEXICO					
					Male					
$/5\ e_x$	1930	3.7601	4.8576	4.9178	4.9028	4.8684	4.8350	4.8045	4.7781	4.7499
$/5\ e_x$	1960	4.4738	4.9653	4.9772	4.9687	4.9527	4.9390	4.9271	4.9116	4.8893
$_5AC_x$	1930-60	.7138	.1077	.0595	.0659	.0844	.1040	.1226	.1335	.1395
$_5RC_x$	1930-60	.5757	.7563	.7231	.6779	.6409	.6304	.6272	.6016	.5575
					Female					
$/5\ e_x$	1930	3.8157	4.8603	4.9241	4.9072	4.8786	4.8507	4.8249	4.8033	4.7821
$/5\ e_x$	1960	4.5177	4.9655	4.9809	4.9750	4.9638	4.9542	4.9445	4.9347	4.9208
$_5AC_x$	1930-60	.7020	.1053	.0568	.0678	.0852	.1034	.1197	.1313	.1387
$_5RC_x$	1930-60	.5928	.7534	.7485	.7306	.7020	.6931	.6833	.6679	.6366
Index	Year(s)	45-49	50-54	55-59	60-64	65-69	70-74	75-79	80-84	
					Male					
$/5\ e_x$	1930	4.7071	4.6410	4.5538	4.4452	4.2971	4.0799	3.7997	3.4825	
$/5\ e_x$	1960	4.8613	4.8195	4.7705	4.7006	4.5956	4.4270	4.1917	3.8921	
$_5AC_x$	1930-60	.1542	.1785	.2167	.2554	.2985	.3470	.3920	.4096	
$_5RC_x$	1930-60	.5265	.4973	.4857	.4604	.4247	.3772	.3266	.2699	
					Female					
$/5\ e_x$	1930	4.7535	4.7043	4.6255	4.4954	4.3469	4.1187	3.8379	3.5170	
$/5\ e_x$	1960	4.9013	4.8711	4.8201	4.7455	4.6333	4.4642	4.2332	3.9333	
$_5AC_x$	1930-60	.1478	.1668	.1946	.2501	.2864	.3455	.3952	.4163	
$_5RC_x$	1930-60	.5995	.5641	.5197	.4957	.4386	.3920	.3401	.2807	

Table A-IV-2 (continued)

Index	Year(s)	0-4	5-9	10-14	15-19	20-24	25-29	30-34	35-39	40-44
		Age Groups								
					NICARAGUA					
					Male					
$/5\ e_x$	1933	3.5980	4.7390	4.8931	4.8898	4.8492	4.8234	4.8061	4.7785	4.7363
$/5\ e_x$	1963	4.2139	4.9125	4.9735	4.9669	4.9436	4.9323	4.9294	4.9202	4.9013
$_5AC_x$	1933-63	.6159	.1735	.0804	.0771	.0944	.1089	.1233	.1416	.1650
$_5RC_x$	1933-63	.4393	.6647	.7524	.6993	.6259	.6166	.6358	.6395	.6258
					Female					
$/5\ e_x$	1933	3.6818	4.7384	4.8873	4.8814	4.8409	4.8119	4.7925	4.7729	4.7512
$/5\ e_x$	1963	4.3085	4.9146	4.9714	4.9652	4.9452	4.9339	4.9298	4.9244	4.9147
$_5AC_x$	1933-63	.6267	.1762	.0841	.0838	.1043	.1220	.1372	.1514	.1635
$_5RC_x$	1933-63	.4754	.6735	.7464	.7065	.6554	.6486	.6615	.6670	.6573

Index	Year(s)	45-49	50-54	55-59	60-64	65-69	70-74	75-79	80-84
					Male				
$/5\ e_x$	1933	4.6781	4.6050	4.5077	4.3741	4.1858	3.9070	3.5248	3.0602
$/5\ e_x$	1963	4.8687	4.8197	4.7482	4.6412	4.4802	4.2405	3.9014	3.4393
$_5AC_x$	1933-63	.1906	.2147	.2405	.2671	.2945	.3335	.3766	.3792
$_5RC_x$	1933-63	.5921	.5436	.4885	.4268	.3617	.3051	.2553	.1955
					Female				
$/5\ e_x$	1933	4.7194	4.6670	4.5894	4.4685	4.2851	4.0167	3.6344	3.1585
$/5\ e_x$	1963	4.8950	4.8606	4.8069	4.7177	4.5713	4.3422	4.0057	3.5514
$_5AC_x$	1933-63	.1756	.1936	.2175	.2492	.2862	.3256	.3713	.3929
$_5RC_x$	1933-63	.6258	.5813	.5297	.4688	.4004	.3311	.2719	.2134

Table A-IV-2 (continued)

Index	Year(s)	0-4	5-9	10-14	15-19	20-24	25-29	30-34	35-39	40-44
					PANAMA					
					Male					
$/5\ e_x$	1930	3.7299	4.7994	4.9304	4.9254	4.8874	4.8646	4.8515	4.8283	4.7907
$/5\ e_x$	1960	4.5397	4.9527	4.9832	4.9782	4.9646	4.9585	4.9570	4.9509	4.9372
$_5AC_x$	1930-60	.8098	.1533	.0528	.0528	.0772	.0938	.1056	.1226	.1465
$_5RC_x$	1930-60	.6376	.7642	.7586	.7083	.6855	.6932	.7107	.7141	.6999
					Female					
$/5\ e_x$	1930	3.8189	4.7912	4.9168	4.9091	4.8715	4.8457	4.8306	4.8160	4.7990
$/5\ e_x$	1960	4.6093	4.9572	4.9848	4.9807	4.9699	4.9641	4.9613	4.9570	4.9487
$_5AC_x$	1930-60	.7904	.1660	.0680	.0716	.0985	.1184	.1307	.1410	.1497
$_5RC_x$	1930-60	.6692	.7950	.8172	.7879	.7659	.7673	.7714	.7661	.7447

Index	Year(s)	45-49	50-54	55-59	60-64	65-69	70-74	75-79	80-84
					Male				
$/5\ e_x$	1930	4.7367	4.6667	4.5712	4.4389	4.2489	3.9653	3.5745	3.0837
$/5\ e_x$	1960	4.9117	4.8714	4.8116	4.7190	4.5769	4.3627	4.0520	3.6151
$_5AC_x$	1930-60	.1750	.2048	.2404	.2801	.3280	.3974	.4775	.5314
$_5RC_x$	1930-60	.6648	.6143	.5606	.4992	.4367	.3841	.3350	.2773
					Female				
$/5\ e_x$	1930	4.7708	4.7214	4.6460	4.5250	4.3396	4.0664	3.6728	3.1685
$/5\ e_x$	1960	4.9322	4.9050	4.8621	4.7909	4.6687	4.4698	4.1700	3.7460
$_5AC_x$	1930-60	.1614	.1836	.2161	.2659	.3291	.4034	.4972	.5776
$_5RC_x$	1930-60	.7041	.6590	.6105	.5598	.4983	.4321	.3746	.3153

Table A-IV-2 (continued)

Index	Year(s)	Age Groups								
		0-4	5-9	10-14	15-19	20-24	25-29	30-34	35-39	40-44
					PARAGUAY					
					Male					
$/5\ e_x$	1932	3.7263	4.7945	4.9259	4.9205	4.8818	4.8585	4.8454	4.8223	4.7851
$/5\ e_x$	1962	4.3553	4.9295	4.9744	4.9685	4.9502	4.9418	4.9399	4.9326	4.9167
$_5AC_x$	1932-62	.6290	.1350	.0486	.0480	.0684	.0833	.0945	.1102	.1317
$_5RC_x$	1932-62	.4939	.6568	.6550	.6042	.5788	.5887	.6114	.6205	.6126
					Female					
$/5\ e_x$	1932	3.8379	4.7931	4.9131	4.9047	4.8673	4.8436	4.8310	4.8176	4.8012
$/5\ e_x$	1962	4.4447	4.9325	4.9734	4.9683	4.9532	4.9449	4.9418	4.9371	4.9284
$_5AC_x$	1932-62	.6068	.1393	.0603	.0636	.0859	.1013	.1108	.1195	.1272
$_5RC_x$	1932-62	.5222	.6735	.6940	.6675	.6472	.6480	.6555	.6552	.6399
Index	Year(s)	45-49	50-54	55-59	60-64	65-69	70-74	75-79	80-84	
					Male					
$/5\ e_x$	1932	4.7306	4.6591	4.5608	4.4216	4.2155	3.8987	3.4402	2.7985	
$/5\ e_x$	1962	4.8889	4.8447	4.7789	4.6800	4.5292	4.3030	3.9797	3.5315	
$_5AC_x$	1932-62	.1583	.1856	.2181	.2583	.3137	.4043	.5395	.7329	
$_5RC_x$	1932-62	.5877	.5445	.4966	.4467	.3999	.3671	.3459	.3329	
					Female					
$/5\ e_x$	1932	4.7724	4.7213	4.6426	4.5130	4.3097	4.0001	3.5318	2.8640	
$/5\ e_x$	1962	4.9106	4.8799	4.8322	4.7521	4.6182	4.4051	4.0875	3.6491	
$_5AC_x$	1932-62	.1382	.1586	.1895	.2390	.3085	.4050	.5557	.7852	
$_5RC_x$	1932-62	.6072	.5691	.5304	.4908	.4469	.4051	.3785	.3676	

Table A-IV-2 (continued)

Index	Year(s)	0-4	5-9	10-14	15-19	20-24	25-29	30-34	35-39	40-44
					VENEZUELA					
					Male					
$/5\ e_x$	1931	3.6652	4.7632	4.9029	4.8985	4.8593	4.8352	4.8205	4.7953	4.7553
$/5\ e_x$	1961	4.6433	4.9797	4.9832	4.9779	4.9700	4.9627	4.9547	4.9422	4.9215
$_5AC_x$	1931-61	.9781	.2165	.0803	.0794	.1108	.1276	.1342	.1468	.1662
$_5RC_x$	1931-61	.7328	.9143	.8274	.7822	.7870	.7740	.7477	.7174	.6793
					Female					
$/5\ e_x$	1931	3.7617	4.7613	4.8953	4.8881	4.8492	4.8220	4.8052	4.7888	4.7705
$/5\ e_x$	1961	4.6873	4.9835	4.9874	4.9837	4.9775	4.9705	4.9622	4.9522	4.9385
$_5AC_x$	1931-61	.9256	.2221	.0922	.0956	.1283	.1486	.1570	.1633	.1679
$_5RC_x$	1931-61	.7475	.9307	.8801	.8544	.8510	.8345	.8062	.7735	.7316

Index	Year(s)	45-49	50-54	55-59	60-64	65-69	70-74	75-79	80-84
					Male				
$/5\ e_x$	1931	4.6987	4.6267	4.5296	4.3957	4.2049	3.9199	3.5276	3.0383
$/5\ e_x$	1961	4.8890	4.8420	4.7743	4.6750	4.5358	4.3400	4.0749	3.7455
$_5AC_x$	1931-61	.1902	.2153	.2448	.2793	.3310	.4201	.5473	.7072
$_5RC_x$	1931-61	.6314	.5767	.5203	.4622	.4163	.3889	.3717	.3605
					Female				
$/5\ e_x$	1931	4.7414	4.6909	4.6141	4.4912	4.3042	4.0290	3.6329	3.1284
$/5\ e_x$	1961	4.9165	4.8807	4.8261	4.7438	4.6252	4.4519	4.2054	3.8842
$_5AC_x$	1931-61	.1751	.1899	.2121	.2526	.3210	.4229	.5725	.7558
$_5RC_x$	1931-61	.6772	.6142	.5494	.4965	.4614	.4355	.4188	.4038

Source: Calculated from Arriaga, New Life Tables.

UNIVERSITY OF CALIFORNIA
2538 Channing Way
Berkeley, California 94720

The Institute of International Studies, in collaboration with International Population and Urban Research (IPUR) and the Department of Demography, announces the publication of a new monograph in its Population Monograph Series:

MORTALITY DECLINE AND ITS DEMOGRAPHIC EFFECTS IN LATIN AMERICA

by

Eduardo E. Arriaga ($3.00)

In an earlier book in this series--New Life Tables for Latin American Populations in the Nineteenth and Twentieth Centuries ($2.75)--Dr. Arriaga has provided basic data for a more accurate history of mortality in Latin America. Now he has used that data to delineate the history itself and to analyze its demographic effects. He has placed particular emphasis on the period 1930-1960 because of its central importance for understanding the demographic evolution of current Latin American populations.

One of the important revelations of this study is that the drop in death rates in Latin America has been even more rapid than was previously thought, providing additional support for the [illegible]

experienced by a major world region. The fall has been so rapid that the populations have had very little time to adjust to the new demographic situation. The result has been a rate of natural increase in excess of anything ever known before in a major region. The rapid decline in mortality has tended to increase fertility, in the sense of the number of offspring per woman. This effect is usually overlooked because the change of the age structure as a consequence of the mortality decline--a change that has enlarged the proportion of people in the childhood ages--has tended to reduce the crude birth rate.

The response of Latin American countries--in terms of fertility--to mortality decline has been substantially different from the European response. European countries have consistently had lower fertility levels than Latin America at various mortality levels. For example, at life expectancy levels of 35, 45, and 55 years, Europe had crude birth rates of 41, 32, and 25 per thousand respectively, while Latin American crude birth rates, at all of these levels, remained close to 44 per thousand. The consequences of this mortality-fertility pattern for the economic and social development of Latin America, as well as the factors that made it impossible for Latin American countries to duplicate the European model, are analyzed in detail in this study.

Dr. Arriaga is a Lecturer in the Department of Demography and a senior member of the staff at IPUR. In addition to the two works he has published in the Population Monograph Series, he has contributed numerous articles to leading demographic journals.

We would appreciate receiving two tear-sheets of any review you might publish, one for the author and the other for our files.

Table A-IV-3

TEMPORARY LIFE EXPECTANCIES FOR 15-YEAR AGE GROUPS FOR SELECTED COUNTRIES: ABSOLUTE AND RELATIVE CHANGES, BY SEX, 1930's TO 1960's

		Age Groups									
		Male					Female				
Index	Year(s)	0-14	15-29	30-34	45-59	60-74	0-14	15-29	30-44	45-59	60-74
					BELGIUM						
$/n\ e_x$	1928-32	13.0749	14.5951	14.4447	13.7353	11.4995	13.4995	14.6193	14.5058	14.0580	12.0422
$/n\ e_x$	1959-63	14.5678	14.8728	14.7672	14.0921	11.7292	14.6640	14.9360	14.8699	14.5141	13.0432
${}_nAC_x$	1928-63	1.4929	.2822	.3225	.3568	.2297	1.2145	.3167	.3641	.4561	1.0010
${}_nRC_x$	1928-63	.7755	.6969	.5808	.2821	.0656	.7833	.8319	.7367	.4842	.3384
					BULGARIA						
$/n\ e_x$	1925-28	11.0704	14.3711	14.2645	13.7008	11.7958	11.3567	14.3485	14.0491	13.8122	12.1945
$/n\ e_x$	1960-62	14.2101	14.8633	14.7670	14.3217	12.2332	14.3265	14.9239	14.8406	14.5191	12.9251
${}_nAC_x$	1925-62	3.1397	.4922	.5025	.6209	.4374	2.9698	.5754	.7915	.7069	.7306
${}_nRC_x$	1925-62	.7990	.7826	.6832	.4779	.1365	.8151	.8832	.8324	.5951	.2604
					CZECHOSLOVAKIA						
$/n\ e_x$	1929-32	12.3213	14.5447	14.3432	13.6430	11.3549	12.6807	14.6050	14.4551	13.9724	11.8083
$/n\ e_x$	1964	14.5588	14.8455	14.7452	14.1945	11.6685	14.6613	14.9423	14.8726	14.5146	12.9934
${}_nAC_x$	1929-64	2.2370	.3008	.4020	.5515	.3136	1.9806	.3373	.4175	.5422	1.1851
${}_nRC_x$	1929-64	.8353	.6607	.6121	.4064	.0860	.8539	.8539	.7662	.5276	.3713

Table A-IV-3 (continued)

		Age Groups									
		Male					Female				
Index	Year(s)	0-14	15-29	30-34	45-59	60-74	0-14	15-29	30-44	45-59	60-74
					ENGLAND AND WALES						
$/_n e_x$	1930-32	13.5085	14.6855	14.5310	13.7939	11.4317	13.8000	14.7139	14.5934	14.1148	12.2510
$/_n e_x$	1963-65	14.5731	14.9187	14.8114	14.1739	11.5742	14.6198	14.9536	14.7982	14.5640	13.0872
$_n AC_x$	1930-65	1.0646	.2332	.2804	.3800	.1425	.8198	.2397	.2048	.4492	.8362
$_n RC_x$	1930-65	.7138	.7415	.5979	.3151	.0399	.6832	.8378	.5037	.5075	.3042
					FRANCE						
$/_n e_x$	1928-33	13.2377	14.5290	14.2293	13.4103	11.0900	13.5300	14.5355	14.4263	13.9463	12.0745
$/_n e_x$	1964	14.5640	14.8518	14.7351	14.1132	11.8373	14.7399	14.9359	14.8891	14.4665	13.3913
$_n AC_x$	1928-64	1.3263	.3228	.5058	.7029	.7473	1.2099	.4004	.4628	.5202	1.3168
$_n RC_x$	1928-64	.7526	.6854	.6563	.4422	.1911	.8231	.8620	.8067	.4937	.4501
					ITALY						
$/_n e_x$	1930-32	12.4988	14.6018	14.4121	13.8675	11.7670	12.6910	14.5939	14.4703	14.1114	12.1925
$/_n e_x$	1960-62	14.2114	14.8586	14.7798	14.2000	12.1581	14.3304	14.9468	14.8489	14.5420	13.1974
$_n AC_x$	1930-62	1.7126	.2568	.3677	.3325	.3911	1.6394	.3529	.3786	.4306	1.0049
$_n RC_x$	1930-62	.6847	.6449	.6254	.2936	.1210	.7100	.8690	.7147	.4846	.3579

Table A-IV-3 (continued)

Index	Year(s)	Male 0-14	Male 15-29	Male 30-34	Male 45-59	Male 60-74	Female 0-14	Female 15-29	Female 30-44	Female 45-59	Female 60-74
		POLAND									
$/n\ e_x$	1931-32	11.8863	14.4063	14.3704	13.4602	11.0206	12.1925	14.5367	14.2414	13.1057	10.8423
$/n\ e_x$	1960-61	14.0371	14.8307	14.7718	14.1147	11.8569	14.1233	14.9248	14.8672	14.4833	12.9448
${}_nAC_x$	1931-61	2.1508	.4244	.4014	.6545	.8363	1.9308	.4081	.6258	1.3776	2.0825
${}_nRC_x$	1931-61	.6908	.7148	.6375	.4251	.2102	.6877	.8809	.8249	.7272	.5009
		SPAIN									
$/n\ e_x$	1930	12.0802	14.4661	14.2131	13.4686	10.9406	12.2725	14.4634	14.3486	13.9795	11.7699
$/n\ e_x$	1960	14.2683	14.8745	14.7500	14.2224	12.2187	14.4159	14.9231	14.8232	14.5223	13.1551
${}_nAC_x$	1930-60	2.1881	.4084	.5369	.7538	1.2781	2.1434	.4597	.4746	.5428	1.3852
${}_nRC_x$	1930-60	.7494	.7649	.6823	.4922	.3148	.7858	.8567	.7286	.5319	.4288
		SWEDEN									
$/n\ e_x$	1921-30	13.6844	14.5710	14.4889	14.0300	12.2419	13.9347	14.6019	14.4973	14.1180	12.5592
$/n\ e_x$	1956-60	14.6456	14.8807	14.8190	14.4042	12.5707	14.8622	14.9513	14.8739	14.5745	13.2086
${}_nAC_x$	1921-60	.9612	.3097	.3301	.3742	.3288	.9275	.3494	.3766	.4565	.6494
${}_nRC_x$	1921-60	.7306	.7219	.6459	.3858	.1192	.8706	.8777	.7492	.5176	.2661
		U.S.A.									
$/n\ e_x$	1929-31	13.7334	14.6675	14.4351	13.6426	11.3763	13.9652	14.7164	14.5021	13.9604	11.9572
$/n\ e_x$	1959-61	14.4798	14.8337	14.7191	13.9029	11.6706	14.5976	14.9306	14.8256	14.4085	13.0320

Table A-IV-3 (continued)

Index	Year(s)	Age Groups									
		Male					Female				
		0-14	15-29	30-34	45-59	60-74	0-14	15-29	30-44	45-59	60-74
${}_nAC_x$	1929-61	.7464	.1662	.2840	.2063	.2943	.6324	.2142	.3055	.4481	1.0748
${}_nRC_x$	1929-61	.5892	.4994	.5027	.1917	.0812	.6111	.7552	.6365	.4310	.3532
					INDIA						
$/n\ e_x$	1921-30	9.1342	13.6903	12.6100	11.2007	9.0621	9.5102	13.2729	12.1329	11.0227	9.3969
$/n\ e_x$	1951-60	11.6156	14.4083	13.7081	12.1180	9.6537	11.5828	14.3771	13.1506	12.0762	10.0987
${}_nAC_x$	1921-60	2.4814	.7180	1.0981	.9173	.5916	2.0726	1.1042	1.0181	1.0535	.7018
${}_nRC_x$	1921-60	.4230	.5482	.4595	.2414	.0996	.3375	.6393	.3550	.2649	.1252
					JAPAN						
$/n\ e_x$	1926-30	11.8286	14.1163	14.2765	13.1095	10.2646	12.0205	13.9767	13.9912	13.4046	11.5016
$/n\ e_x$	1959-60	14.3374	14.8091	14.7026	14.0772	11.6271	14.4498	14.8823	14.7714	14.3750	12.7734
${}_nAC_x$	1926-60	2.5088	.6928	.4261	.9677	1.3625	2.4293	.9056	.7802	.9704	1.2718
${}_nRC_x$	1926-60	.7911	.7840	.5889	.5119	.2877	.8153	.8850	.7734	.6082	.3635
					TAIWAN						
$/n\ e_x$	1936-40	11.3280	14.3732	13.7620	12.3881	9.6340	11.5785	14.4522	14.0154	13.3847	11.1928
$/n\ e_x$	1959-60	13.8947	14.8129	14.6053	13.8699	11.1729	13.9469	14.8439	14.6864	14.2709	12.3829
${}_nAC_x$	1936-60	2.5667	.4397	.8433	1.4818	1.5389	2.3684	.3917	.6710	.8862	1.1901
${}_nRC_x$	1936-60	.6990	.7015	.6812	.5673	.2868	.6922	.7150	.6815	.5486	.3126

Source: Calculated from United Nations, Demographic Yearbook 1953, Tables 18 and 19, and Demographic Yearbook 1966, Tables 21 and 23.

APPENDIX IV

Table A-IV-4

LIFE EXPECTANCIES AT BIRTH IN SELECTED LATIN AMERICAN COUNTRIES: 1930's AND 1960's

Year	Male	Female	Difference Between Sexes
	BRAZIL		
1930	33.10	34.15	1.05
1960	54.03	57.04	3.01
P.I.[a]	20.96	22.89	1.96
	CHILE		
1930	34.55	37.75	1.20
1960	54.18	58.71	4.53
P.I.	19.63	22.96	3.33
	COSTA RICA		
1933	42.54	44.54	2.00
1963	62.15	65.03	2.88
P.I.	19.61	20.49	.88
	EL SALVADOR		
1931	29.71	29.61	-.10
1961	52.63	55.57	2.94
P.I.	22.92	25.96	3.04
	GUATEMALA		
1934	26.40	26.28	-.12
1964	49.26	53.27	4.01
P.I.	22.86	26.99	4.13
	HONDURAS		
1931	33.76	34.87	1.11
1961	52.63	55.57	2.94
P.I.	18.87	20.70	1.83

[a]P.I. means period increase.

Table A-IV-4 (continued)

Year	Male	Female	Difference Between Sexes
	MEXICO		
1930	33.02	34.70	1.68
1960	56.37	59.58	3.21
P.I.[a]	23.35	24.88	1.53
	NICARAGUA		
1933	30.76	31.80	1.04
1963	50.52	53.29	2.77
P.I.	19.76	21.49	1.73
	PANAMA		
1930	35.54	36.23	.69
1960	59.75	63.18	3.43
P.I.	24.21	26.95	2.74
	PARAGUAY		
1932	34.94	36.18	1.24
1962	54.25	57.24	2.99
P.I.	19.31	21.06	1.75
	VENEZUELA		
1931	32.45	33.60	1.15
1961	61.19	64.69	3.50
P.I.	28.74	31.09	2.35

[a]P.I. means period increase.

Source: Calculated from Arriaga, New Life Tables.

APPENDIX IV

Table A-IV-5

TEMPORARY LIFE EXPECTANCIES IN CHILDBEARING AGE GROUPS IN SELECTED LATIN AMERICAN COUNTRIES: ABSOLUTE AND RELATIVE CHANGES, BY SEX, 1930's TO 1960's

Index	Year(s)	Male 15-44	Male 20-49	Female 15-44	Female 20-49
		BRAZIL			
$/n\ e_x$	1930	25.1111	24.3474	24.8093	24.1208
$/n\ e_x$	1960	28.1478	27.8067	28.2421	27.9622
$_nAC_x$	1930-60	3.0367	3.4593	3.4328	3.8414
$_nRC_x$	1930-60	.6211	.6120	.6613	.6354
		CHILE			
$/n\ e_x$	1930	25.5920	24.8266	25.2953	24.6161
$/n\ e_x$	1960	28.3400	27.8064	28.7989	28.4517
$_nAC_x$	1930-60	2.7480	2.9797	3.5036	3.8357
$_nRC_x$	1930-60	.6234	.5760	.7447	.7124
		COSTA RICA			
$/n\ e_x$	1933	26.7135	26.1717	26.6253	26.1618
$/n\ e_x$	1963	29.1186	28.8669	29.3226	29.0953
$_nAC_x$	1933-63	2.4051	2.6952	2.6973	2.9335
$_nRC_x$	1933-63	.7318	.7040	.7993	.7653
		EL SALVADOR			
$/n\ e_x$	1931	24.5593	23.6865	24.2927	23.4098
$/n\ e_x$	1961	28.2455	27.9027	28.3405	28.0593
$_nAC_x$	1931-61	3.6863	4.2162	4.0478	4.6496
$_nRC_x$	1931-61	.6775	.6678	.7092	.7055
		GUATEMALA			
$/n\ e_x$	1934	24.2389	23.1251	23.3692	22.3673
$/n\ e_x$	1964	27.6419	27.2174	27.7144	27.4057
$_nAC_x$	1934-64	3.4030	4.0923	4.3452	5.0384
$_nRC_x$	1934-64	.5907	.5953	.6553	.6601

Table A-IV-5 (continued)

Index	Year(s)	Age Groups			
		Male		Female	
		15-44	20-49	15-44	20-49
		HONDURAS			
$/n\ e_x$	1931	25.2729	24.5270	24.9719	24.3080
$/n\ e_x$	1961	28.1263	27.7405	28.2016	27.8858
$_nAC_x$	1931-61	2.8534	3.2135	3.2297	3.5779
$_nRC_x$	1931-61	.6036	.5872	.6423	.6286
		MEXICO			
$/n\ e_x$	1930	25.2087	24.2757	25.5830	24.7987
$/n\ e_x$	1960	28.1362	27.6262	28.5684	28.2043
$_nAC_x$	1930-60	2.9275	3.3505	2.9854	3.4057
$_nRC_x$	1930-60	.6110	.5853	.6759	.6548
		NICARAGUA			
$/n\ e_x$	1933	24.7402	23.9090	24.4937	23.7379
$/n\ e_x$	1963	27.9435	27.5132	27.9887	27.6334
$_nAC_x$	1933-63	3.2033	3.6043	3.4950	3.8955
$_nRC_x$	1933-63	.6090	.5917	.6347	.6221
		PANAMA			
$/n\ e_x$	1930	25.9352	25.1559	25.4517	24.7670
$/n\ e_x$	1960	28.6972	28.4230	28.8644	28.6391
$_nAC_x$	1930-60	2.7620	3.2671	3.4127	3.8721
$_nRC_x$	1930-60	.6795	.6745	.7503	.7399
		PARAGUAY			
$/n\ e_x$	1932	25.7656	24.9847	25.3817	24.7390
$/n\ e_x$	1962	28.1959	27.8540	28.2824	28.0017
$_nAC_x$	1932-62	2.4303	2.8693	2.9007	3.2628
$_nRC_x$	1932-62	.5739	.5721	.6281	.6202
		VENEZUELA			
$/n\ e_x$	1931	25.0743	24.2828	24.7756	24.0719
$/n\ e_x$	1961	28.7785	28.4337	29.0377	28.7486
$_nAC_x$	1931-61	3.7042	4.1509	4.2620	4.6767
$_nRC_x$	1931-61	.7520	.7260	.8158	.7889

Source: Calculated from Arriaga, New Life Tables.

Table A-IV-6

DEATH RATES FOR AGE 15 TO 29, BY SEX, IN SELECTED COUNTRIES: 1960's

(Per hundred thousand)

		Male			Female			
Country	Year	Total	Accidents	Total Minus Accidents	Total	Pregnancies	Accidents	Total Minus Accidents and Pregnancies
LATIN AMERICA								
Chile[a]	1960	362.19	167.98	194.22	261.68	43.53	30.79	185.36
Costa Rica	1961	150.69	69.15	81.54	108.16	29.90	8.91	69.35
El Salvador	1961	385.53	209.14	174.39	233.77	26.80	25.91	181.06
Guatemala	1961	483.83	98.22	385.61	522.00	45.00	15.85	461.15
Mexico	1960	339.59	149.67	189.92	272.17	34.80	19.48	217.89
Nicaragua	1961	282.46	119.86	162.59	218.81	35.60	12.04	171.17
Panama	1961	196.97	71.49	125.48	213.07	38.53	24.94	149.61
Venezuela	1961	196.79	110.37	86.42	145.36	19.55	24.39	101.43
EUROPE[b]								
Belgium	1961	133.22	83.99	49.23	53.83	2.53	19.79	31.51
Bulgaria	1961	127.27	64.89	62.38	79.81	5.21	14.52	60.08
Czechoslovakia	1961	147.71	97.46	50.25	55.58	3.61	17.18	34.79
England and Wales	1961	98.44	57.21	41.23	47.64	2.81	12.47	32.36
France	1961	135.05	84.87	50.18	59.62	3.34	19.37	36.91
Italy	1961	132.52	76.62	55.90	64.76	6.49	11.33	46.94
Poland	1961	160.10	91.97	68.13	78.76	3.09	15.31	60.36
Portugal	1961	160.15	65.52	94.63	90.19	8.80	12.22	69.17
Sweden	1961	100.43	65.86	34.57	46.70	.80	15.39	30.51
Switzerland	1961	134.00	96.25	37.75	48.76	2.98	18.50	27.28
U.S.A.	1961	155.31	106.34	48.97	67.68	3.93	24.52	39.23

[a]For ages 15-34.

[b]The United States was included because of characteristic similiarity.

Source: Calculated from World Health Organization, Epidemiological Yearbook 1961.

Table A-IV-7

DEATH RATES FOR AGE 30 TO 44, BY SEX, IN SELECTED COUNTRIES: 1960's

(Per hundred thousand)

Country	Year	Male			Female			
		Total	Accidents	Total Minus Accidents	Total	Pregnancies	Accidents	Total Minus Accidents and Pregnancies
LATIN AMERICA								
Chile[a]	1960	778.36	300.13	478.23	507.72	57.09	26.22	424.41
Costa Rica	1961	280.42	92.40	188.02	292.77	49.15	10.69	232.93
El Salvador	1961	681.34	266.70	414.63	483.87	43.99	21.01	418.87
Guatemala	1961	875.78	144.25	731.54	866.11	69.20	25.82	771.09
Mexico	1960	693.45	224.59	468.86	502.84	49.80	23.67	429.37
Nicaragua	1961	526.01	156.92	369.10	438.95	62.05	12.03	364.87
Panama	1961	338.55	103.64	234.92	347.31	41.43	21.94	283.94
Venezuela	1961	401.05	135.60	265.46	344.07	31.87	23.44	288.77
EUROPE[b]								
Belgium	1961	241.42	81.96	159.46	141.47	3.46	18.39	119.62
Bulgaria	1961	347.96	86.13	261.83	244.58	4.91	20.43	219.24
Czechoslovakia	1961	246.29	103.61	142.68	138.63	2.65	21.52	114.46
England and Wales	1961	202.75	46.80	155.95	148.67	3.11	16.73	128.83
France	1961	355.38	130.98	224.40	150.15	4.91	21.49	123.75
Italy	1961	236.79	65.92	170.87	148.98	11.19	11.07	126.72
Poland	1961	253.72	79.80	173.92	174.44	4.26	16.57	153.61
Portugal	1961	338.92	79.20	259.72	199.39	17.25	13.84	168.30
Sweden	1961	182.17	69.19	112.98	113.45	2.00	14.99	96.46
Switzerland	1961	235.20	100.04	135.16	136.13	4.99	25.48	105.66
U.S.A.	1961	307.01	95.92	211.09	187.06	4.53	28.07	154.45

[a]For ages 35-44.

[b]The United States was included because of characteristic similarity.

Source: Same as Table A-IV-6.

P A R T   I I I

THE EFFECTS AND CONSEQUENCES OF RAPID MORTALITY DECLINE

Chapter V

THE EFFECT OF MORTALITY DECLINE ON AGE STRUCTURE AND POPULATION GROWTH

The age structure of a population as well as its growth is determined by three parameters: fertility, migration, and mortality. If migration is nil--a closed population--the age structure depends mainly on fertility; moderate mortality changes do not greatly modify it. This fact has been illustrated by theoretical models as well as by actual European populations. The historical demographic trends in Europe show the populations to be much more affected by the decline of fertility than by the gradual mortality decline over a long period.[1] Nevertheless, when mortality falls suddenly and continuously at a very fast rate during a considerable number of years--as it has in Latin America since the 1930's--some noticeable effects on the age structure of the population can be expected. Also, as noted in previous chapters, the unprecedented mortality decline in Latin America has produced very rapid population growth.

This chapter examines the effect of mortality decline on the age structure and on the total growth of the population. An explanation of the methodology used, however, is first in order.

Methodology Used

The stable population theory helps in understanding how fertility and mortality changes produce variations in the age

---

[1]F. Lorimer, "Dynamics of Age Structure in a Population with Initially High Fertility and Mortality," Population Bulletin No. 1 (New York: United Nations, December 1951): 31-41; United Nations, "The Cause of the Aging of Populations: Declining Mortality or Declining Fertility?" Population Bulletin No. 4 (New York, December 1954): 30-38; United Nations, The Aging of Populations and Its Economic and Social Implications (New York, 1956); A. Sauvy, "Le Vieillissement des populations et l'allongement de la vie," Population, No. 4 (1954): 675-682; V.G. Valaoras, "Patterns of Aging of Human Populations," The Social and Biological Challenge of Our Aging Population (New York: Columbia University Press, 1950); L. Feraud, "A propos du vieillissement d'une population," Proceedings of the World Population Conference, Vol. III (Rome: United Nations, 1954).

structure of a population. According to this theory, any change in the intrinsic birth rate will change the age structure of the stable population. This is easily understood when it is remembered that the proportion of the stable population at age "zero" is the intrinsic birth rate: $C(0) = b$. Hence, if b changes, the proportion at age zero $C(0)$ will change too, and because the summation of the $C(x)$ must be one, another age (or other ages) also has (or have) to change.[2]

---

[2]We have referred to intrinsic birth rates rather than fertility for the following reasons: Constant age-specific fertility rates with a changing proportional age structure--at least in the reproductive ages--will produce, in general, different intrinsic birth rates. If the intrinsic birth rate changes, the age structure will change also. On the other hand, with constant intrinsic birth rates and changing proportional age structure, at least in the reproductive ages (because of mortality), the age-specific fertility rates must change, but this change of fertility will not affect the proportional age structure distribution. If the intrinsic birth rate does not change, fertility--whether it does or does not change--will not affect the proportional age distribution.

The statement about proportional age structure of a stable population $C(x)$, the intrinsic birth rate b, and the age-specific fertility rate $m(x)$ can be explained by analyzing the following well-known equations:

$$b = \int_{\alpha}^{\beta} C(x)\, m(x)\, dx \qquad \text{(I)}$$

$$C(x) = b\, e^{-rx}\, l_x \qquad \text{(II)}$$

where x is age, r is the intrinsic growth rate, and α and β are the lower and upper limits of the female reproductive ages. Let us analyze three cases:

Case A. It is possible to have infinite different sets of age-specific fertility rates--$m(x)$--with constant $C(x)$ between the reproductive ages α to β under the condition that b in equation (I) does not change. Under the previous condition, equation (II) will not change if l_x doesn't change.

Case B. It is possible to have infinite different sets of $C(x)$ between ages α and β with constant $m(x)$'s that will satisfy the conditions of same values b in equation (I). Equation (II) will change because of change of mortality--l_x--and also in r.

Case C. It is possible to have infinite different combination sets of $C(x)$ and $m(x)$ which will satisfy the equation (I) for a constant value of b. As in Case B, equation (II) will

The effect of a change in mortality, on the other hand, is somewhat different. Generally, a change in the intrinsic death rate--or in the probability of surviving--will change the age structure, but there is an important exception. The exception occurs when the probability of being alive changes in the same proportion for all ages, or when the force of mortality changes in the same absolute quantity for all ages.[3]

This change of mortality which does not affect the proportional age distribution--the "neutral change of mortality," as Keyfitz calls it--can be deduced as follows: If the intrinsic birth rate remains constant and the proportion of population in each age does not have to change, and if we assign "prime" values, signifying those rates after the mortality change, we can write

---

vary because of the changes in l_x and r.

The demographic restrictions to these cases are:

(1) $C(x+n) \gtreqless C(x)$, because

$$C(x+n) = C(x) \frac{l_{x+n}}{l_x} e^{-rn}$$

where the quotients $\frac{l_{x+n}}{l_x}$ for positive values of n cannot be greater than one--that is, $l_{x+n} \leqq l_x$.

(2) $0 \leqq m(x) \leqq \lambda$

The maximum limit of any age-specific fertility rates is λ because of the limitation of the time needed from conception to birth.

(3) $r \geqq 0$.

[3]The effect of mortality and fertility on the age structure of the population has been widely explained in several articles and books. See, for example: United Nations, The Aging of Populations; Ansley Coale, "The Effects of Changes in Mortality and Fertility on Age Composition," Milbank Memorial Fund Quarterly, XXXIV, No. 1 (January 1956): 79-114; Nathan Keyfitz, Introduction to the Mathematics of Population (Reading, Mass.: Addison-Wesley Publishing Co., 1968), pp. 185-194--esp. the "neutral change of mortality," p. 187; Leo Goodman, "On the Age-Sex Composition of the Population that Would Result from Given Fertility and Mortality Conditions," Demography, 4, No. 2 (1967): 423-442.

$$b = b' \qquad \text{(V-1)}$$

$$C(x) = C'(x) \qquad \text{(V-2)}$$

Because of the change in mortality, the intrinsic death rate and the intrinsic growth rate will change, as well as the probability of surviving from birth to any particular age. In symbols

$$d = d' + \delta \qquad \text{(V-3)}$$

$$r = r' - \delta \qquad \text{(V-4)}$$

$$1_x \neq 1'_x \qquad \text{(V-5)}$$

where 1_x is the function of a life table where 1_o is one (in other words, 1_x is Lotka's p(a)).[4]

Keeping this in mind, we can write

$$C(x) = b\, 1_x\, e^{-rx} = b'\, 1'_x\, e^{-r'x} = C'(x) \qquad \text{(V-6)}$$

But because $b = b'$ and $r' = r + \delta$,

$$1'_x = e^{\delta x}\, 1_x \qquad \text{(V-7)}$$

This means that the proportional age distribution of the new stable population--C'(x)--which has the same intrinsic birth rate as the old, will not change if the two sets of 1_x functions (from the previous and changed life tables) maintain an exponential relationship in relation to age. A further step will clarify this. The probability of being alive one year more is

$$p_x = \frac{1_{x+1}}{1_x} \qquad \text{(V-8)}$$

Therefore, the new probability of being alive after the change of mortality, according to (V-6), will be

$$p'_x = p_x\, e^{\delta} \qquad \text{(V-9)}$$

This is the result presented by Coale: the new stable population will have the same proportional age distribution after the

---

[4] Alfred J. Lotka, Theorie analytique des associations biologiques (Paris: Hermann & Cie., Editeurs, 1939).

mortality change if the previous and new probabilities of being alive differ in equal proportion for all ages.[5] In addition, by taking the natural logarithm, multiplying by -1, and using the relationship between the force of mortality and the probability of being alive $\mu_x = -\ln p_x$, we obtain from (V-7)

$$\mu'_x = \mu_x - \delta \qquad \text{(V-10)}$$

where δ is Keyfitz's "neutral change of mortality."[6] This means that the force of mortality should change with the same absolute value in all ages.

It is now possible to determine the maximum change in a life expectancy in order to have the possibility of a "neutral change of mortality." Because p_x cannot be more than one, and μ_x cannot be negative, δ has a limit. The limit is obviously the minimal value in the μ_x set. The life expectancy at birth is

$$\overset{o}{e}_o = \int_o^{\omega} l_x \, dx \qquad \text{(V-11)}$$

After the change of mortality, the new life expectancy would be

$$\overset{o}{e}'_o = \int_o^{\omega} l'_x \, dx = \int_o^{\omega} e^{\delta x} l_x \, dx \qquad \text{(V-12)}$$

An approximation of the new life expectancy is obtained by

$$\overset{o}{e}'_o \approx \sum_o^{\omega} e^{\delta(x+.5)} L_x \qquad \text{(V-13)}$$

with L_x and δ (the minimum value of μ_x) values from the life table before the mortality change. The lower the life expectancy, the greater the value of μ_x and hence the greater the chance that the change of the life expectancy would allow the possibility of a "neutral change of mortality."

In Latin America, the levels of life expectancy in the 1930's were low. Therefore, the possibility did exist then of having a "neutral change of mortality." Whether such a possibility existed from 1930 to 1960 can be established by analyzing the

---

[5] Coale, "Changes in Mortality and Fertility."

[6] Keyfitz, Mathematics of Population.

situation of the country with the lowest life expectancy level in the 1930's--Guatemala--which in 1934 had a male life expectancy at birth of 26.3 years.[7] The minimum value of μ_x, which is also the value of δ in formula (V-13), was .009214 for age 14. With formula (V-13) the maximum possible life expectancy change allowing for the possibility of a neutral mortality change can be determined for a country with a mortality level as high as Guatemala's in 1934. There could have been a neutral mortality change only if life expectancy at birth had remained under 34.12 years--that is, a change from the 1930's level in Guatemala of less than 30 percent.

In all Latin American countries, a greater than 30 percent change in life expectancy occurred during the 1930-1960 period; thus it is certain that the age structure of the population has been affected by the mortality decline. The results obtained in the previous chapter also lead to such a conclusion. As the reader will remember, the absolute increase in the number of years to be lived (the ${}_nAC_x$ index in Table IV-2) differed for all age groups. Therefore, there is no doubt that the large and rapid mortality decline registered in Latin America has affected the age distributions of these populations.

Stable population theory could help in an analysis of the changes in the age structure resulting from this mortality decline. I prefer, however, to use other procedures, partly because of the lack of accurate information needed for the calculation of stable populations in the 1930's, and partly because I am interested in the actual changes in the actual populations rather than the differences between two stable populations with the 1930 and 1960 demographic characteristics of these countries.

Procedure Applied to Latin American Population

In order to discover how the enumerated populations of the 1960's have been affected by mortality decline during the period from 1930 to 1960, we must compare the actually enumerated 1960 populations with those 1960 populations as they would have been had mortality remained constant since the 1930's. These latter populations will be labeled hypothetical "A" populations, in order to distinguish them from other hypothetical populations used in Chapter VIII (to be known as hypothetical "B" populations).

The procedure to be applied depended on the availability of data in the countries under consideration. For the period

---

[7] This figure is taken from an interpolated life table for 1934.

under study, several difficulties had to be surmounted: (a) there was no reliable information on age-specific fertility rates;[8] (b) the populations were exposed to some extent to international migration, and information about that movement was inaccurate; (c) not all the countries to be studied took a census in the 1930's, and those censuses taken were frequently not comparable with those of the 1960's, because the completeness of the enumerations was not the same.[9]

In order to overcome these difficulties, the following procedure was used: (a) the 1960's census populations were first corrected for underenumeration in ages under 5 and then smoothed; (b) the populations for each sex were rejuvenated to the 1930's by using the reciprocals of the survivor ratios obtained from the available life tables;[10] (c) the 1930's rejuvenated populations were used as the basis for projecting the population up to the 1960's with constant mortality in order to obtain hypothetical "A" populations.

This procedure avoids the informational problems of age-specific fertility rates and international migration. Age-specific fertility rates are not needed because during the process of rejuvenation from the 1960's to the 1930's, 5-year period birth rates and 5-year period masculinity at birth rates were calculated.[11] With respect to migration, immigrants under age 30 in the 1960's are assumed to be native-born citizens of the country to which they have emigrated, immigrants 30 years of age and over are assumed to have entered the country before the 1930's, and all emigrants to other countries--regardless of age--are ignored. Because international migration was insignificant for most of the countries during the 1930-1960 period, these assumptions will not affect the analysis.[12]

---

[8]We should know the actual age-specific fertility rates in order to be sure that changes in the age distribution of the population were not due to fertility.

[9]See census figures in Arriaga, New Life Tables.

[10]Ibid.

[11]Constant age-specific fertility rates with age structure changing because of mortality will produce a different birth rate, which will again affect the age structure. By using the birth rates, we avoid any effects due to this circular interaction (see footnote 2).

[12]Only Venezuela experienced considerable immigration and Paraguay, emigration, during the 1950-1960 decade. For Venezuela, the rejuvenation-projection process was applied to the native

If the rejuvenated populations in the 1930's are projected by using the same mortality levels as in the rejuvenation process (which are assumed to be the actual levels) and also the same period's birth rates and masculinity at birth (estimated in the rejuvenation process), the hypothetical "A" population in the 1960's will be, obviously, the same as the enumerated population. Therefore, if instead of projecting the population from the 1930's to the 1960's with the actual mortality, the projections are made with mortality levels of the 1930's held constant (using the same estimated period birth rates and masculinity at birth found during the rejuvenation process), the difference between the hypothetical "A" and the actual populations will be due exclusively to the decline of mortality. (The deduction of all formulae used in the rejuvenation process as well as those used in order to obtain the hypothetical "A" population are given in Appendix V. The results for the eleven countries together are given in Table V-1 and for each particular country in Table A-V-1.)

The Effect of the Mortality Decline on the Age Structures

The mortality decline in Latin American countries has clearly affected the age structures of these populations. In order to present a general pattern of these changes, we will first consider the changes in the mean ages of the populations and later the changes in the age structures themselves.

Changes in the Mean Ages of the Populations. The actual mean ages of the Latin American populations have tended to decline. For instance, the average mean age for 10 countries has dropped from 23.2 in the 1930's to 22.1 in the 1960's (see Table V-2). This change of 1.1 has resulted from changes in mortality, fertility, and international migration. However, because these mean ages were calculated by using census information, a part of this difference could be due to faulty enumeration, age misreporting, and other census errors. The effect of mortality change alone can be obtained by comparing the mean ages of the actual 1960's populations with the mean ages of the hypothetical "A" populations. On the average, the reduction of mortality tended to make these populations younger by .7 years. In every country the mortality effect was to reduce the mean age of the population within a range between .5 years (Brazil) and 1.3 years (Venezuela), as can be seen in Table V-3. The mean age reduction because of mortality decline is greater than the actual change in

---

population in 1961. The results obtained--the effect of the mortality decline on the age structure--were exactly the same as those found by using the whole population.

Table V-1

ACTUAL AND HYPOTHETICAL "A" POPULATIONS IN ELEVEN LATIN AMERICAN COUNTRIES, BOTH SEXES: 1960's

(thousands)

Age Group	Actual Population	Hypothetical "A" Population	Differences: Absolute (1)-(2)	Differences: Relative (3)÷(1)	Percent Distribution Column (3)
	(1)	(2)	(3)	(4)	(5)
Total	136,937.9	109,869.3	27,068.6	19.8	100.0
0- 4	24,557.0	17,645.3	6,911.7	28.1	25.5
5- 9	20,279.9	14,844.3	5,435.6	26.8	20.1
10-14	16,600.8	13,072.3	3,528.5	21.3	13.0
15-19	13,885.1	11,600.2	2,284.9	16.5	8.4
20-24	11,570.5	10,047.7	1,522.8	13.2	5.6
25-29	9,832.7	8,725.6	1,107.1	11.3	4.1
30-34	8,384.7	7,468.4	916.3	10.9	3.4
35-39	7,129.9	6,278.7	851.2	11.9	3.1
40-44	5,964.9	5,165.1	799.8	13.4	3.0
45-49	4,963.8	4,219.6	744.2	15.0	2.7
50-54	4,007.2	3,337.6	669.6	16.7	2.5
55-59	3,211.1	2,609.3	601.8	18.7	2.2
60-64	2,480.6	1,953.1	527.5	21.3	1.9
65-69	1,817.1	1,373.0	444.1	24.4	1.6
70-74	1,182.6	842.1	340.5	28.8	1.3
75-79	593.8	387.5	206.3	34.7	.8
80-84	283.4	163.0	120.4	42.5	.4
85+	192.8	136.5	56.3	29.2	.2
0-14	61,437.7	45,561.9	15,875.8	25.8	58.7
15-49	61,731.6	53,505.3	8,226.3	13.3	30.4
50-64	9,698.9	7,900.0	1,798.9	18.5	6.6
65+	4,069.7	2,902.1	1,167.6	28.7	4.3

Source: Appendix V, Table A-V-1.

Table V-2

MEAN AGES OF TOTAL CENSUS POPULATIONS FOR SELECTED LATIN AMERICAN COUNTRIES: 1930-1960

Country	1930		1960		Difference
	Census Year	Mean Age of Total Population	Census Year	Mean Age of Total Population	
Brazil	1930[a]	22.5	1960	22.5	.0
Chile	1930	24.9	1960	24.8[b]	.1
Costa Rica	1927	23.1	1963	21.3[c]	1.8
El Salvador	1930	23.4	1961	21.9	1.5
Guatemala	1940	22.4	1964	21.6	.8
Honduras	1930	22.3	1961	21.1	1.2
Mexico	1930	24.0	1960	22.1	1.9
Nicaragua	1940	22.8	1963	21.1	1.7
Panama	1930	23.2	1960	23.3	-.1
Venezuela	1936	23.5	1961	20.9	2.6
Non-Weighted Average		23.2		22.1	1.1

[a]Interpolated between 1920 and 1940.

[b]_Poblacion del Pais, Caracteristicas Basicas de la Poblacion, Censo 1960_ (Santiago, Chile, 1964).

[c]Costa Rica, Ministerio de Industria y Commerce, _Censo de Poblacion_ (Abril 1966), p. 380.

Source: Calculated from census populations.

Table V-3

MEAN AGE OF ACTUAL AND HYPOTHETICAL "A" POPULATIONS IN LATIN AMERICAN COUNTRIES: 1960's

Country	Actual Populations			Hypothetical "A" Populations			Differences		
	Total	Male	Female	Total	Male	Female	Total	Male	Female
Brazil	22.52	22.47	22.56	23.06	23.17	22.95	.54	.70	.39
Chile	24.79	24.39	25.18	25.43	25.08	25.76	.64	.69	.58
Costa Rica	21.33	21.23	21.43	22.07	21.96	22.18	.74	.73	.75
El Salvador	21.92	21.59	22.24	23.12	22.76	23.47	1.20	1.17	1.23
Guatemala	21.60	21.55	21.65	22.83	22.79	22.87	1.23	1.24	1.22
Honduras	21.06	20.82	21.30	21.63	21.39	21.87	.57	.57	.57
Mexico	22.11	21.80	22.41	23.04	22.76	23.31	.93	.96	.90
Nicaragua	21.17	20.72	21.61	21.91	21.48	22.32	.74	.76	.71
Panama	23.35	23.50	23.19	24.19	24.38	24.00	.84	.88	.81
Paraguay	22.79	22.32	23.25	23.39	22.96	23.81	.60	.64	.56
Venezuela	20.90	20.45	21.34	22.18	21.83	22.54	1.28	1.38	1.20
Average[a]	22.41	22.27	22.55	23.14	23.09	23.18	.73	.82	.63

[a]The values for the average pertain to the population of the eleven countries combined.

Sources: Table V-4 and Appendix V, Table A-V-1

four countries and smaller in six. In those countries where the mean age change due to the mortality decline was greater than the actual change--Brazil, Chile, Guatemala, and Panama--other factors such as fertility, international migration, or completeness of the censuses counteracted the change due to mortality. In the other six countries--Costa Rica, El Salvador, Honduras, Mexico, Nicaragua, and Venezuela--those factors combined with mortality to bring about the decline in the mean age of the population.

Changes in the Age Structures. Of the 27 million people alive in all the eleven countries in the 1960's who would not have been alive if there had not been a mortality decline since the 1930's, 16 million--59 percent--were under age 15 (see Table V-1). Ten million were in the 15 to 64 age group and only one million in the 65 and over age group.[13] It seems that, in absolute terms, the older the age, the smaller the number of persons alive because of the mortality decline.

However, if those persons alive due to mortality decline are measured in relation to the total number of persons alive in each age group in the 1960's, the picture alters. These relative increases have a "U"-shaped trend: youth and the aged benefitted most from mortality reduction. The results for both sexes together for the eleven countries combined are:

	Populations (thousands)		Differences	
Age Group	Actual	Hypothetical "A"	Absolute (1)-(2)	Percent (3)÷(1)
	(1)	(2)	(3)	(4)
0-15[a]	61,437.7	45,561.9	15,875.8	25.8
15-49	61,731.6	53,505.3	8,226.3	13.3
50-64	9,698.9	7,900.0	1,798.9	18.5
65+	4,069.7	2,902.1	1,167.6	28.7
Total	136,937.9	109,869.3	27,068.6	19.8

[a] See Table V-1 for the trend by 5-year age groups.

[13] This agrees with the analysis made in Chapter IV, where we saw that the younger ages benefitted more by the mortality decline. Another advantage of using the temporary life expectancies in the analysis of mortality decline is illustrated here: they give an idea of how the population would be affected by mortality decline.

As a consequence of the distribution of the "saved" people, the proportional age group distribution of the population was affected. The percentages of the total population in ages under 15 and 65 and over increased while the percentage in ages 15 to 64 decreased, as shown below for the population (both sexes) of the eleven Latin American countries combined.

Age Group	Percent Population Distribution: Actual	Percent Population Distribution: Hypothetical "A"	Difference
Total	100.0	100.0	
0-14[a]	44.8	41.5	3.3
15-49	45.1	48.7	-3.6
50-64	7.1	7.2	-.1
65+	3.0	2.6	.4

[a]See Table V-4 for 5-year age groups.

The same pattern of percentage change is repeated in every country. The largest changes occurred in Guatemala and the smallest in Brazil (see details by country in Appendix V, Table A-V-1).

The mortality decline almost identically affected the proportional age group distribution of each sex toward a younger age distribution. Both distributions have almost the same changes as those already considered for both sexes; thus it is not necessary to repeat them. (The changes for the eleven countries combined can be seen in Table V-4 and for individual countries in Appendix V, Table A-V-1.) The proportion of people in each age group who were alive in the 1960's because of the mortality decline, compared to all those who were alive in the same ages, has the same "U"-shaped pattern in each sex, and is practically identical to that of both sexes together (see Appendix V, Table A-V-2).

The Effect of the Mortality Decline on Total Population Growth

Had mortality remained constant from the 1930's, one out of every five persons enumerated in the eleven Latin American

Table V-4

PROPORTIONAL AGE DISTRIBUTION OF ACTUAL AND HYPOTHETICAL "A" POPULATIONS IN ELEVEN LATIN AMERICAN COUNTRIES: 1960's

(percentages)

Age Group	Total		Male		Female	
	Actual	Hypothetical "A"	Actual	Hypothetical "A"	Actual	Hypothetical "A"
Total	100.000	100.000	100.000	100.000	100.000	100.000
0- 4	17.933	16.060	18.313	16.436	17.555	15.680
5- 9	14.810	13.511	15.001	13.744	14.619	13.275
10-14	12.123	11.898	12.135	11.956	12.111	11.839
15-19	10.140	10.558	10.052	10.497	10.227	10.620
20-24	8.449	9.145	8.284	8.871	8.614	9.422
25-29	7.180	7.942	7.021	7.673	7.339	8.214
30-34	6.123	6.798	6.018	6.597	6.227	7.001
35-39	5.207	5.715	5.147	5.579	5.266	5.852
40-44	4.356	4.701	4.359	4.657	4.352	4.745
45-49	3.625	3.841	3.648	3.852	3.602	3.829
50-54	2.926	3.038	2.955	3.093	2.898	2.982
55-59	2.345	2.375	2.370	2.456	2.320	2.292
60-64	1.811	1.778	1.826	1.862	1.797	1.692
65-69	1.327	1.250	1.328	1.316	1.326	1.183
70-74	0.864	0.766	0.845	0.801	0.882	0.732
75-79	0.434	0.353	0.402	0.354	0.465	0.352
80-84	0.207	0.148	0.182	0.143	0.232	0.153
85+	0.141	0.124	0.114	0.113	0.168	0.136
0-14	44.865	41.469	45.449	42.136	44.285	40.794
15-49	45.080	48.699	44.530	47.727	45.627	49.683
50-64	7.083	7.190	7.151	7.411	7.015	6.967
65+	2.972	2.641	2.870	2.726	3.074	2.555

Source: Calculated from Appendix V, Table A-V-2.

countries in the 1960's--that is, 27 million Latin Americans--would not have been alive. The percentage of additional people in each country who were alive in the 1960's ranges from 17.0 percent in Brazil to 31.7 percent in Guatemala (see Table V-5). The population of 110 million people which would have been enumerated in the 1960's under the conditions of constant mortality since the 1930's was actually reached in the 1950's. In approximately 20 years (1930-1950), mortality decline accounted for a growth in population which would otherwise have taken 30 years (1930-1960). Its effect can further be appreciated by comparing the actual populations of the eleven Latin American countries with their hypothetical populations, had mortality declined at the same rate as in European countries at the same mortality level. From the 1930's to the 1960's, the population of the Latin American countries would have risen to only 115 million, instead of to the 137 million that were enumerated. (For similar comparisons for other years, see Table V-6.)

The sharp decline of mortality beginning in the 1930's accelerated Latin American population growth to a very high rate in a very short period of time. Instead of a growth rate of 14 per thousand in the 1960's for the eleven countries, which would have occurred under mortality conditions constant since the 1930's, the actual rate jumped to 32 per thousand. Under mortality conditions of the 1930's the population would have doubled in 50 years, while under mortality conditions of the 1960's, doubling will occur in only 22. In other words, during a 50-year period, when a population with the 1930's mortality rate would double, a population with the 1960's mortality rate would quadruple.

In the eleven Latin American countries combined, females benefitted more than males by the mortality decline. There was an excess of 76 females for each thousand males among those who were alive in the 1960's due to the mortality decline since the 1930's (see Table V-7).

Although general trends were the same, each country was affected to a different degree. The number of persons of each sex "saved" because of the mortality decline depended on the total number of each sex, the age structure, the sex ratio at birth, the change in mortality, and the level at which mortality change occurred. Since these factors were not the same in each country, the changes between sexes produced by the mortality decline differed. In three countries--Costa Rica, Mexico, and Venezuela--the number of males who survived because of the mortality decline was slightly greater than the number of females; in the rest of the countries, the situation was reversed. Brazil, the most populated country, had the greatest difference between sexes: one million more females than males, though in relative terms the difference was not far from parity. The extreme cases were Venezuela, where 982 females were alive for each thousand

Table V-5

ACTUAL AND HYPOTHETICAL "A" POPULATIONS IN SELECTED LATIN AMERICAN COUNTRIES: 1960's

(thousands)

Country	Year	Actual Populations			Hypothetical "A" Populations			Difference as Percentage of Actual		
		Total	Male	Female	Total	Male	Female	Total	Male	Female
		136,930.8	68,306.7	68,624.1	109,868.5	55,273.2	54,595.3	19.8	19.0	20.4
Brazil	1960	71,776.2	35,806.6	35,969.6	59,608.9	30,205.6	29,403.3	17.0	15.6	18.3
Chile	1960	7,410.6	3,633.8	3,776.8	6,024.9	2,957.8	3,067.1	18.6	18.6	18.8
Costa Rica	1963	1,355.0	678.8	676.2	1,108.4	554.6	553.8	18.2	18.3	18.1
El Salvador	1961	2,578.7	1,271.4	1,307.3	1,768.6	879.6	889.0	31.4	30.8	32.0
Guatemala	1964	4,280.7	2,135.7	2,145.0	2,917.3	1,466.3	1,451.0	31.7	31.3	32.4
Honduras	1961	1,881.3	937.3	944.0	1,561.1	778.1	783.0	17.0	17.0	17.1
Mexico	1960	35,691.2	17,811.6	17,879.6	27,940.5	13,915.3	14,025.2	21.7	21.9	21.6
Nicaragua	1963	1,532.5	756.7	775.8	1,195.4	589.8	605.6	22.0	22.1	21.9
Panama	1960	1,011.5	515.0	496.5	791.3	405.2	386.1	21.8	21.3	22.2
Paraguay	1962	1,803.8	893.3	910.5	1,460.4	722.8	737.7	19.0	19.1	19.0
Venezuela	1961	7,608.5	3,865.7	3,742.8	5,491.7	2,797.6	2,694.1	27.8	27.6	28.0

Source: From Appendix V, Table A-V-1.

Table V-6

ACTUAL AND HYPOTHETICAL "A" POPULATIONS OF ELEVEN LATIN AMERICAN COUNTRIES: 1930-2020[a]

(thousands)

	Populations		
Year	Actual[b]	Hypothetical "A"[c]	European Mortality Trend[d]
1930	71,048.8	71,048.8	71,048.8
1950	102,986.5	94,419.0	96,227.7
1960	136,937.9	109,868.5	115,205.4
1990	355,445.3	168,727.3	223,624.3
2020	922,665.7	259,118.1	567,628.4

[a]The countries included are Brazil, Chile, Costa Rica, El Salvador, Guatemala, Honduras, Mexico, Nicaragua, Panama, Paraguay, and Venezuela.

[b]Actual populations for 1930, 1950, and 1960. Beyond 1960 it is assumed that the population will grow at an annual geometric growth rate of 31.8 per thousand.

[c]From 1930 to 1960, projected population with constant 1930 mortality. Beyond 1960 the growth rate of the population is assumed to be constant at the 1960 rate--14.3 per thousand.

[d]From 1930 to 1960, the 1930 population is projected using actual crude birth rates and crude death rates declining at the pace registered in Europe when this region had the Latin American mortality level. Beyond 1960, a constant crude birth rate of 44 per thousand and declining crude death rates following the European trend are assumed.

Table V-7

SEX AND AGE GROUPS IN ACTUAL AND HYPOTHETICAL "A" POPULATIONS IN ELEVEN LATIN AMERICAN COUNTRIES: 1960's[a]

(thousands)

Age Group	Male Populations			Female Populations			Ratio Female to Male Difference
	Actual	Hypothetical "A"	Difference (1)-(2)	Actual	Hypothetical "A"	Difference (4)-(3)	(6)÷(3)
	(1)	(2)	(3)	(4)	(5)	(6)	(7)
Total	68,310.1	55,272.8	13,037.3	68,627.8	54,596.5	14,031.3	1.076
0-14	31,046.2	23,289.6	7,756.6	30,391.5	22,272.3	8,119.2	1.047
15-49	30,418.6	26,379.9	4,038.7	31,313.0	27,125.4	4,187.6	1.037
50-64	4,884.9	4,096.4	788.5	4,814.0	3,803.6	1,010.4	1.281
65+	1,960.4	1,506.9	453.5	2,109.3	1,395.2	714.1	1.575

[a]For individual countries, see Appendix V, Table A-V-3.

Source: Appendix V, Table A-V-2.

males, and Brazil, where there were 1,172 females per thousand males (see Appendix V, Table A-V-3).

Summary

The very rapid mortality decline in Latin America since the 1930's has altered the age structure of the population toward a younger age configuration, with the proportion of those under age 15 now considerably larger. The mortality decline without a change of fertility has also produced a rapid population growth. If demographic conditions of the 1960's continue in the future, the Latin American population will double every 22 years.

Appendix V

Census Correction

The corrected populations for Chile, Costa Rica, Mexico, and Venezuela in the 1960's were taken from a previous study.[1] For the other seven countries considered here, the population aged 0 to 5 was estimated by using the number of births during the 5-year period before the census and the survivor ratio for births. The male population in ages 0-4 would be

$$^{m}N^{t}_{0-4} = h \cdot B^{t-5,t} \cdot {}^{m}P^{t-5,t} \qquad \text{(A-V-1)}$$

where h is masculinity at birth,[2] and

$$^{m}P_{b}^{t-5,t} = \frac{{}_{5}^{m}L_{x}}{5 \cdot {}^{m}l_{0}} \qquad \text{(A-V-2)}$$

where the superscript m refers to males. The total number of births--$B^{t-5,t}$--was found by using the equation

$$B^{t-5,t} = 2.5\ (b^{t-5} \cdot N^{t-5} + b^{t} \cdot N^{t}) \qquad \text{(A-V-3)}$$

where b^{t} and b^{t-5} are estimated birth rates for the census year t and 5 years earlier, t-5; N^{t} is the census population; and N^{t-5} is an interpolated total population using census figures at time t-5. The same procedure was applied for females. (The corrected 1960 populations can be seen in Appendix V, Table A-V-1.)

The survivor ratios for the period 1930 to 1960 for all ages were calculated by interpolating the 5-year survivor ratios from the life tables available for each country, using polynomial functions in the procedure explained in Chapter IV, Appendix IV.

---

[1] Arriaga, New Life Tables.

[2] Total male births per hundred births.

APPENDIX V

Rejuvenation

If ${}^{m}N^{t}_{x,x+5}$ is the male population in the age group x,x+5 at time t (${}^{f}N^{t}_{x,x+5}$ for females), and ${}^{m}P^{t,t+5}_{x,x+5}$ the survivor ratio for those males x,x+5 years old at the beginning of the period t,t+5 (${}^{f}P^{t,t+5}_{x,x+5}$ for females), then the number of people alive 5 years before is

$$ {}^{m}N^{t}_{x,x+5} = \frac{{}^{m}N^{t+5}_{x+5,x+10}}{{}^{m}P^{t,t+5}_{x,x+5}} \qquad \text{(A-V-4)} $$

By successively repeating this operation, we obtained the population for each sex in the 1930's starting from the population in the 1960's for the eleven Latin American countries.

The total number of births of males for every 5-year period was obtained as follows:

$$ {}^{m}B^{t,t+5} = \frac{{}^{m}N^{t+5}_{0-5}}{{}^{m}P^{t,t+5}_{b}} \qquad \text{(A-V-5)} $$

The same method was applied for females. The addition of male and female births gave the total number of births $B^{t,t+5}$. The masculinity at birth for each 5-year period was calculated as

$$ h^{t,t+5} = \frac{{}^{m}B^{t,t+5}}{B^{t,t+5}} \qquad \text{(A-V-6)} $$

Birth rates for each 5-year period were estimated as

$$ b^{t,t+5} = \frac{B^{t,t+5}}{\int_{0}^{5} N^{t+i} di} \qquad \text{(A-V-7)} $$

Using the hypothesis that the population grows geometrically--$N^{t+i} = N^{t} . e^{ri}$--and integrating the denominator, the following is obtained:

$$ b^{t,t+5} = \frac{r^{t,t+5} . B^{t,t+5}}{N^{t+5} - N^{t}} \qquad \text{(A-V-8)} $$

where $r^{t,t+5}$ is the average annual geometric rate of instant growth of the total population for every 5-year period. That is,

$$r^{t,t+5} = \frac{1}{5} \ln \frac{N^{t+5}}{N^{t}} \qquad \text{(A-V-9)}$$

Projection from the 1930's to the 1960's

The projected population from the 1930's to the 1960's, which is called the hypothetical "A" population and differs from the actual enumerated population at the end of the period only because it was exposed to a different mortality, was obtained by using (a) the rejuvenated population in the 1930's as the base population for the projection, (b) the 5-year period birth rates and masculinity estimated in the process of rejuvenation, and (c) constant survivor ratios for the 1930's. The difference between the enumerated and the hypothetical "A" populations is due exclusively to the change of mortality during the 30-year period.[3] For each 5-year interval of the period, the hypothetical "A" population for ages 5 and over was determined as

$$^{m}N^{t+5}_{x+5,x+10} = {}^{m}N^{t}_{x,x+5} \cdot {}^{m}P^{t,t+5}_{x,x+5} \qquad \text{(A-V-10)}$$

for males as well as females.

In order to obtain the population under age 5, the total number of births during each 5-year period is needed. These births cannot be obtained directly by transforming formula (A-V-8), because neither the total population at time t+5 nor the period growth rate is known.[4] Hence, some modification for formula (A-V-8) is necessary in order to obtain the total number of births during each 5-year period. The total population in two age groups at time t+5 can be expressed as

$$N^{t+5} = N^{t+5}_{-5} + N^{t+5}_{5+} \qquad \text{(A-V-11)}$$

[3]As we saw before, if instead of constant survivor ratios, such as those of the 1930's, the projection was made using the actual mortality throughout the period (that of the life tables), we would obtain exactly the same populations as the enumerated ones.

[4]Total population and growth rates were obtained in the rejuvenation process with changing actual mortality. Now, with constant 1930's mortality, both figures will change.

Formula (A-V-10) allows us to obtain N_{5+}^{t+5}. The population under age 5 can also be expressed as a function of the births and survivor ratios as

$$N_{-5}^{t+5} = B^{t,t+5} \cdot P_b^{t,t+5} \qquad \text{(A-V-12)}$$

Therefore,

$$N^{t+5} = B^{t,t+5} \cdot P_b^{t,t+5} + N_{5+}^{t+5} \qquad \text{(A-V-13)}$$

The annual growth rate of formula (A-V-8) could be expressed as in formula (A-V-9), but the logarithmic function presents some problems in solving formula (A-V-8) for the total number of births. Hence, in order to simplify the equation, the annual growth rate is expressed by the relation

$$r^{t,t+5} = .4 \frac{N^{t+5} - N^t}{N^{t+5} + N^t} \qquad \text{(A-V-14)}$$

The results obtained by using equations (A-V-14) and (A-V-9) are almost the same.[5]

By replacing the growth rate of formula (A-V-8) with formula (A-V-14), cancelling, replacing N^{t+5} of formula (A-V-8) with formula (A-V-13), and making the necessary algebraic manipulations, the total number of births during the 5-year period is obtained:

---

[5]The difference between formula (A-V-9) and (A-V-14) is very small when the population is growing slowly, i.e., when the growth rate is low. In Latin American countries, the growth rates were low due to the fact that mortality was maintained at 1930's levels. Because fertility remained practically unchanged during the 30-year period, the growth rates were close to the values observed in the 1930's, which were small. For instance, in Costa Rica, the Latin American country with the highest growth rate in the 1930's, the geometric rate--formula (A-V-9)--was .018721, while the rate from formula (A-V-14) was .018708. From 1930 to 1935, from an initial population of 555.4 thousand, a total population of 609,899 is obtained using the geometric growth rate of .018721, while a figure of 609,859 is obtained with a rate of .018708. The population growth rates for the rest of the Latin American countries were much lower than Costa Rica's rate; thus the differences in results from the two equations are even less.

APPENDIX V

$$B^{t,t+5} = \frac{b^{t,t+5}\ (N_{5+}^{t+5} + N^{t})}{.4 - b^{t,t+5}\ .\ P_{b}^{t,t+5}} \qquad \text{(A-V-15)}$$

All the symbols on the right side are now known except the survivor ratio for both sexes, $P_{b}^{t,t+5}$, which is calculated from the survivor ratios for each sex as

$$P_{b}^{t,t+5} = h^{t,t+5}\ .\ {}^{m}P_{b}^{t,t+5} + (1-h^{t,t+5})\ .\ {}^{f}P_{b}^{t,t+5} \qquad \text{(A-V-16)}$$

where $h^{t,t+5}$ is the masculinity at birth for each 5-year period.

The total number of births of each sex during the 5-year period is obtained by using the previously calculated masculinity at birth.

$${}^{m}B^{t,t+5} = h^{t,t+5}\ .\ B^{t,t+5} \qquad \text{(A-V-17)}$$

$${}^{f}B^{t,t+5} = (1-h^{t,t+5})\ .\ B^{t,t+5} \qquad \text{(A-V-18)}$$

By multiplying the number of male and female births by the respective survivor ratios at birth, the population under age 5 for each of the sexes is found, and thus all the age groups for the year t+5 are obtained, under the same "actual" period birth rates, the same period masculinity at birth, and constant mortality as at time t. The hypothetical "A" population was projected with constant mortality from the 1930's to the 1960's by successively making all these steps. The comparison of the actual population in the 1960's with the hypothetical "A" population gives the effect of mortality decline on the age structure of Latin American populations; calculations made for the eleven countries are given in Table A-V-1.

APPENDIX V

Table A-V-1

ABSOLUTE AND PROPORTIONAL AGE GROUP DISTRIBUTION IN ACTUAL AND HYPOTHETICAL "A" POPULATIONS IN LATIN AMERICAN COUNTRIES: 1960's

BRAZIL: 1960

Age Group	Populations (thousands)			
	Male		Female	
	Actual	Hypothetical "A"	Actual	Hypothetical "A"
Total	35,808.2	30,205.6	35,971.4	29,403.3
0- 4	6,392.1	4,924.3	6,163.4	4,537.8
5- 9	5,317.3	4,220.3	5,242.2	3,962.0
10-14	4,306.7	3,639.1	4,366.3	3,524.8
15-19	3,589.4	3,164.5	3,716.3	3,149.4
20-24	2,988.0	2,632.8	3,150.4	2,814.2
25-29	2,551.6	2,270.5	2,693.9	2,448.1
30-34	2,204.4	1,959.3	2,289.8	2,088.6
35-39	1,895.3	1,668.0	1,934.7	1,747.1
40-44	1,614.4	1,407.1	1,593.8	1,410.3
45-49	1,351.1	1,174.2	1,309.3	1,122.1
50-54	1,088.1	950.0	1,037.1	850.0
55-59	865.2	761.9	819.3	634.8
60-64	653.5	577.7	621.6	452.2
65-69	468.0	410.3	451.8	307.7
70-74	293.7	251.9	295.1	186.2
75-79	130.7	107.0	151.5	87.3
80-84	58.3	44.2	74.9	38.2
85+	40.4	42.4	60.0	42.5
	Percentages			
0-14	44.727	42.322	43.846	40.896
15-49	45.225	47.265	46.393	50.266
50-64	7.280	7.580	6.889	6.588
65+	2.768	2.833	2.873	2.251

APPENDIX V

Table A-V-1 (continued)

CHILE: 1960

	Populations (thousands)			
	Male		Female	
Age Group	Actual	Hypothetical "A"	Actual	Hypothetical "A"
Total	3,634.5	2,957.8	3,776.6	3.067.1
0- 4	582.0	420.2	575.8	420.6
5- 9	492.4	352.7	489.0	351.7
10-14	417.3	329.5	423.2	333.4
15-19	357.0	307.6	368.2	315.3
20-24	301.2	270.8	318.0	283.2
25-29	261.8	238.0	279.7	250.3
30-34	230.1	208.8	247.1	219.6
35-39	202.6	182.1	217.2	190.9
40-44	178.5	157.7	188.8	163.9
45-49	153.9	132.8	162.6	139.4
50-54	129.3	108.5	136.5	115.2
55-59	106.6	86.6	113.2	93.4
60-64	85.4	66.7	91.2	72.7
65-69	63.3	47.2	69.5	52.6
70-74	37.7	26.4	47.6	33.5
75-79	21.9	14.1	26.3	16.8
80-84	8.3	4.7	13.0	7.2
85+	5.2	3.6	9.7	7.6
	Percentages			
0-14	41.043	37.271	39.401	36.048
15-49	46.364	50.636	47.175	50.947
50-64	8.840	8.849	9.027	9.169
65+	3.753	3.244	4.398	3.836

APPENDIX V

Table A-V-1 (continued)

COSTA RICA: 1963

Age Group	Populations (thousands)			
	Male		Female	
	Actual	Hypothetical "A"	Actual	Hypothetical "A"
Total	679.2	554.6	676.5	553.8
0- 4	137.1	102.6	133.0	100.2
5- 9	110.5	83.8	107.1	81.6
10-14	84.7	67.8	84.4	67.6
15-19	67.7	56.9	68.3	57.3
20-24	53.0	46.3	54.6	47.4
25-29	43.9	39.4	45.2	40.2
30-34	36.8	33.5	37.8	33.9
35-39	31.3	28.3	32.0	28.6
40-44	26.6	23.8	26.8	23.8
45-49	22.3	19.6	22.4	19.7
50-54	18.3	15.7	18.2	15.8
55-59	14.7	12.2	14.7	12.6
60-64	11.5	9.2	11.5	9.6
65-69	8.6	6.6	8.7	6.9
70-74	5.9	4.3	5.8	4.4
75-79	3.4	2.3	3.3	2.3
80-84	1.5	.9	1.5	.9
85+	1.4	1.3	1.2	1.1
	Percentages			
0-14	48.925	45.832	47.967	45.024
15-49	41.461	44.684	42.439	45.313
50-64	6.552	6.697	6.563	6.857
65+	3.062	2.787	3.030	2.806

APPENDIX V

Table A-V-1 (continued)

EL SALVADOR: 1961

Age Group	Populations (thousands)			
	Male		Female	
	Actual	Hypothetical "A"	Actual	Hypothetical "A"
Total	1,271.7	879.6	1,307.7	889.0
0- 4	247.6	147.3	242.0	141.2
5- 9	200.8	121.0	198.3	115.5
10-14	156.8	103.1	157.2	100.0
15-19	126.9	91.0	130.1	90.7
20-24	102.0	78.8	108.5	81.9
25-29	85.0	69.8	92.3	74.5
30-34	72.4	61.1	79.3	65.9
35-39	61.5	51.2	67.2	54.9
40-44	51.9	41.8	55.5	43.7
45-49	43.4	33.5	45.9	34.8
50-54	35.2	25.8	36.8	26.9
55-59	28.5	19.8	29.7	20.7
60-64	22.7	14.8	23.6	15.6
65-69	16.7	10.2	17.6	10.8
70-74	10.5	5.9	11.5	6.4
75-79	5.2	2.6	5.8	2.8
80-84	2.6	1.1	3.4	1.3
85+	2.0	.9	3.0	1.3
	Percentages			
0-14	47.590	42.218	45.691	40.128
15-49	42.707	48.568	44.261	50.224
50-64	6.794	6.868	6.890	7.107
65+	2.909	2.346	3.158	2.540

APPENDIX V

Table A-V-1 (continued)

GUATEMALA: 1964

Age Group	Populations (thousands)			
	Male		Female	
	Actual	Hypothetical "A"	Actual	Hypothetical "A"
Total	2,135.7	1,466.3	2,145.1	1,451.0
0- 4	410.5	238.7	403.7	233.4
5- 9	333.9	193.7	330.8	191.3
10-14	262.0	168.1	262.4	166.9
15-19	214.5	154.1	217.0	152.8
20-24	174.4	137.7	181.2	138.8
25-29	146.7	123.7	153.1	124.0
30-34	125.4	107.7	129.3	106.1
35-39	106.5	89.5	108.6	87.0
40-44	89.7	72.2	89.2	69.0
45-49	74.0	56.4	73.2	54.6
50-54	58.2	41.6	57.9	41.6
55-59	46.4	31.0	46.0	31.6
60-64	36.3	22.6	36.0	23.5
65-69	26.4	15.3	26.1	15.8
70-74	16.9	8.9	16.5	9.2
75-79	7.8	3.6	7.3	3.6
80-84	3.4	1.3	4.0	1.6
85+	2.7	.2	2.8	.3
	Percentages			
0-14	47.123	40.956	46.473	40.771
15-49	43.602	50.550	44.362	50.464
50-64	6.597	6.493	6.522	6.664
65+	2.678	2.001	2.643	2.101

APPENDIX V

Table A-V-1 (continued)

HONDURAS: 1961

Age Group	Populations (thousands)			
	Male		Female	
	Actual	Hypothetical "A"	Actual	Hypothetical "A"
Total	937.4	778.1	944.0	783.0
0- 4	186.2	141.3	179.4	136.5
5- 9	151.3	117.6	148.6	115.5
10-14	118.5	98.0	117.7	97.1
15-19	95.9	83.1	97.0	83.8
20-24	77.0	68.7	80.0	71.0
25-29	63.7	57.7	67.0	60.1
30-34	53.2	48.3	56.0	50.1
35-39	44.5	40.0	46.6	41.3
40-44	36.8	32.5	37.7	33.0
45-49	30.2	26.2	30.7	26.6
50-54	24.1	20.4	24.4	20.8
55-59	19.2	15.8	19.4	16.3
60-64	14.9	11.9	15.1	12.4
65-69	10.6	8.2	10.9	8.6
70-74	6.5	4.8	7.1	5.4
75-79	2.6	1.8	3.5	2.5
80-84	1.3	.8	1.6	1.0
85+	.9	.7	1.3	1.1
	Percentages			
0-14	48.645	45.872	47.214	44.582
15-49	42.810	45.835	43.962	46.728
50-64	6.209	6.196	6.239	6.321
65+	2.336	2.097	2.585	2.370

APPENDIX V

Table A-V-1 (continued)

MEXICO: 1960

Age Group	Populations (thousands)			
	Male		Female	
	Actual	Hypothetical "A"	Actual	Hypothetical "A"
Total	17,812.7	13,915.3	17,880.4	14,025.2
0- 4	3,407.5	2,373.7	3,238.7	2,270.1
5- 9	2,716.0	1,898.6	2,618.4	1,836.4
10-14	2,209.3	1,672.7	2,181.4	1,654.6
15-19	1,812.5	1,470.5	1,829.2	1,484.6
20-24	1,468.3	1,252.4	1,529.2	1,301.4
25-29	1,223.7	1,077.0	1,291.3	1,132.8
30-34	1,025.6	909.5	1,080.6	955.1
35-39	864.0	756.8	907.7	792.5
40-44	719.6	620.1	745.5	639.9
45-49	602.0	511.1	620.7	524.5
50-54	495.5	413.9	511.6	425.2
55-59	404.5	329.6	416.9	338.8
60-64	322.8	254.0	330.9	261.1
65-69	241.5	180.5	248.7	189.2
70-74	161.4	112.1	169.0	120.2
75-79	82.5	52.2	91.8	59.4
80-84	38.2	21.1	44.7	25.5
85+	17.8	9.5	24.1	13.8
	Percentages			
0-14	41.077	44.957	42.723	46.780
15-49	48.704	44.765	47.410	43.316
50-64	7.309	7.043	7.169	6.865
65+	2.911	3.234	2.698	3.039

APPENDIX V

Table A-V-1 (continued)

NICARAGUA: 1963

Age Group	Populations (thousands)			
	Male		Female	
	Actual	Hypothetical "A"	Actual	Hypothetical "A"
Total	756.4	589.8	775.8	605.6
0- 4	152.8	107.6	146.4	103.3
5- 9	123.5	88.4	120.9	86.6
10-14	96.1	73.6	96.9	74.1
15-19	77.3	62.6	79.9	64.5
20-24	61.7	52.3	65.7	55.3
25-29	50.7	44.3	54.9	47.6
30-34	42.1	37.2	45.6	40.0
35-39	35.0	30.6	37.7	32.7
40-44	28.7	24.6	30.4	25.9
45-49	23.4	19.4	24.8	20.7
50-54	18.5	14.9	19.7	16.0
55-59	14.9	11.6	15.9	12.6
60-64	11.7	8.8	12.7	9.7
65-69	8.7	6.3	9.6	7.0
70-74	5.6	3.8	6.6	4.6
75-79	2.8	1.8	3.8	2.4
80-84	1.7	1.0	2.5	1.4
85+	1.2	1.0	1.8	1.4
	Percentages			
0-14	49.233	45.716	46.945	43.582
15-49	42.160	45.962	43.697	47.326
50-64	5.962	5.985	6.226	6.325
65+	2.644	2.338	3.132	2.767

APPENDIX V

Table A-V-1 (continued)

PANAMA: 1960

Age Group	Populations (thousands)			
	Male		Female	
	Actual	Hypothetical "A"	Actual	Hypothetical "A"
Total	515.1	405.2	496.5	386.1
0- 4	86.1	58.7	83.7	57.4
5- 9	73.3	51.3	71.6	50.1
10-14	61.1	46.3	59.9	45.1
15-19	51.7	42.0	50.8	40.7
20-24	43.1	36.9	42.4	35.6
25-29	37.1	33.1	36.1	31.4
30-34	32.0	29.2	30.7	27.1
35-39	27.9	25.2	26.2	22.9
40-44	24.2	21.3	22.2	19.0
45-49	20.4	17.5	18.6	15.6
50-54	16.4	13.5	15.0	12.4
55-59	13.2	10.5	12.0	9.6
60-64	10.0	7.5	9.2	7.1
65-69	7.5	5.3	7.0	5.1
70-74	5.5	3.6	5.2	3.5
75-79	3.7	2.2	3.5	2.1
80-84	1.3	.7	1.4	.7
85+	.6	.4	1.0	.6
	Percentages			
0-14	42.807	38.593	43.343	39.537
15-49	45.894	50.623	45.720	49.828
50-64	7.688	7.776	7.291	7.527
65+	3.611	3.008	3.646	3.108

APPENDIX V

Table A-V-1 (continued)

PARAGUAY: 1962

Age Group	Populations (thousands)			
	Male		Female	
	Actual	Hypothetical "A"	Actual	Hypothetical "A"
Total	893.3	722.8	910.5	737.7
0- 4	161.7	117.4	157.4	115.3
5- 9	137.1	101.5	133.5	99.6
10-14	113.3	89.8	110.5	87.8
15-19	93.6	78.8	92.6	77.6
20-24	73.7	64.8	75.6	65.8
25-29	60.5	54.8	63.6	56.6
30-34	49.5	45.4	53.6	48.0
35-39	41.5	37.7	45.8	40.6
40-44	35.2	31.3	39.3	34.5
45-49	29.9	26.0	33.3	28.8
50-54	25.2	21.3	27.4	23.4
55-59	21.2	17.3	22.5	18.8
60-64	18.1	14.2	17.8	14.5
65-69	14.1	10.6	14.0	10.9
70-74	9.7	6.9	10.5	7.7
75-79	5.1	3.3	7.2	4.9
80-84	2.4	1.4	3.4	2.0
85+	1.5	.4	2.5	.6
	Percentages			
0-14	46.132	42.712	44.086	41.051
15-49	42.975	46.862	44.349	47.712
50-64	7.220	7.298	7.435	7.691
65+	3.672	3.127	4.130	3.547

APPENDIX V

Table A-V-1 (continued)

VENEZUELA: 1961

Age Group	Populations (thousands)			
	Male		Female	
	Actual	Hypothetical "A"	Actual	Hypothetical "A"
Total	3,865.9	2,797.6	3,743.3	2,694.1
0- 4	746.1	452.8	723.8	444.7
5- 9	591.3	367.6	572.1	357.6
10-14	463.3	320.5	451.8	312.2
15-19	379.7	291.0	369.5	281.4
20-24	316.7	261.9	305.8	250.0
25-29	271.6	233.0	259.3	218.4
30-34	239.7	206.1	223.7	187.9
35-39	205.9	174.1	190.2	156.9
40-44	172.3	141.9	157.8	127.7
45-49	141.3	112.5	130.4	103.5
50-54	109.7	83.9	104.1	80.8
55-59	84.4	61.4	82.7	62.2
60-64	60.7	41.8	63.4	45.6
65-69	41.5	26.7	46.3	31.1
70-74	24.1	14.1	30.2	18.4
75-79	8.7	4.5	15.4	8.1
80-84	5.0	2.1	9.0	3.8
85+	3.9	1.9	7.8	3.8
	Percentages			
0-14	46.579	40.781	46.689	41.368
15-49	44.678	50.774	43.723	49.213
50-64	6.591	6.687	6.684	7.000
65+	2.152	1.758	2.904	2.419

APPENDIX V

Table A-V-2

ACTUAL AND HYPOTHETICAL "A" POPULATIONS IN ELEVEN LATIN AMERICAN COUNTRIES COMBINED: 1960's

(thousands)

Age Group	Actual Population	Hypothetical "A" Population	Differences: Absolute (1)-(2)	Differences: Relative (3)÷(1)	Percent Distribution Column (3)
	(1)	(2)	(3)	(4)	(5)
			Male		
Total	68,310.1	55,272.8	13,037.3	19.1	100.0
0- 4	12,509.7	9,084.6	3,425.1	27.4	26.3
5- 9	10,247.4	7,596.5	2,650.9	25.9	20.3
10-14	8,289.1	6,608.5	1,680.6	20.3	12.9
15-19	6,866.2	5,802.1	1,064.1	15.5	8.2
20-24	5,659.1	4,903.4	755.7	13.4	5.8
25-29	4,796.3	4,241.3	555.0	11.6	4.3
30-34	4,111.2	3,646.1	465.1	11.3	3.6
35-39	3,516.0	3,083.5	432.5	12.3	3.3
40-44	2,977.9	2,574.3	403.6	13.6	3.1
45-49	2,491.9	2,129.2	362.7	14.6	2.8
50-54	2,018.5	1,709.5	309.0	15.3	2.4
55-59	1,618.8	1,357.7	261.1	16.1	2.0
60-64	1,247.6	1,029.2	218.4	17.5	1.7
65-69	906.9	727.2	179.7	19.8	1.4
70-74	577.5	442.7	134.8	23.3	1.0
75-79	274.4	195.4	79.0	28.8	.6
80-84	124.0	79.3	44.7	36.0	.3
85+	77.6	62.3	15.3	19.7	.1
0-14	31,046.2	23,289.6	7,756.6	25.0	59.5
15-49	30,418.6	26,379.9	4,038.7	13.3	31.0
50-64	4,884.9	4,096.4	788.5	16.1	6.0
65+	1,960.4	1,506.9	453.5	23.1	3.5

APPENDIX V

Table A-V-2 (continued)

Age Group	Actual Population	Hypothetical "A" Population	Differences		Percent Distribution Column (3)
			Absolute (1)-(2)	Relative (3)÷(1)	
	(1)	(2)	(3)	(4)	(5)
			Female		
Total	68,627.8	54,596.5	14,031.3	20.4	100.0
0- 4	12,047.3	8,560.7	3,486.6	28.9	24.8
5- 9	10,032.5	7,247.8	2,784.7	27.8	19.8
10-14	8,311.7	6,463.8	1,847.9	22.2	13.2
15-19	7,018.9	5,798.1	1,220.8	17.4	8.7
20-24	5,911.4	5,144.3	767.1	13.0	5.5
25-29	5,036.4	4,484.3	552.1	11.0	3.9
30-34	4,273.5	3,822.3	451.2	10.6	3.2
35-39	3,613.9	3,195.2	418.7	11.6	3.0
40-44	2,987.0	2,590.8	396.2	13.3	2.8
45-49	2,471.9	2,090.4	381.5	15.4	2.7
50-54	1,988.7	1,628.1	360.6	18.1	2.6
55-59	1,592.3	1,251.6	340.7	21.4	2.4
60-64	1,233.0	923.9	309.1	25.1	2.2
65-69	910.2	645.8	264.4	29.0	1.9
70-74	605.1	399.4	205.7	34.0	1.5
75-79	319.4	192.1	127.3	39.9	.9
80-84	159.4	83.7	75.7	47.5	.5
85+	115.2	74.2	41.0	35.6	.3
0-14	30,391.5	22,272.3	8,119.2	26.7	57.9
15-49	31,313.0	27,125.4	4,187.6	13.4	29.8
50-64	4,814.0	3,803.6	1,010.4	21.0	7.2
65+	2,109.3	1,395.2	714.1	33.9	5.1

Table A-V-3

COMPARISON OF SEX AND AGE GROUPS IN ACTUAL AND HYPOTHETICAL "A" POPULATIONS IN LATIN AMERICAN COUNTRIES: 1960's

	Populations (thousands)						
	Male			Female			Ratio of Female to Male Difference (6)÷(3)
	Actual	Hypothetical "A"	Difference (1)-(2)	Actual	Hypothetical "A"	Difference (4)-(5)	
Age Group	(1)	(2)	(3)	(4)	(5)	(6)	(7)
BRAZIL: 1960							
Total	35,808.2	30,205.6	5,602.6	35,971.4	29,403.3	6,568.1	1.172
0-14	16,016.1	12,783.7	3,232.4	15,771.9	12,024.6	3,747.3	1.159
15-49	16,194.2	14,276.6	1,917.6	16,688.2	14,779.8	1,908.4	.995
50-64	2,606.8	2,289.5	317.3	2,478.0	1,937.1	540.9	1.705
65+	991.1	855.8	135.3	1,033.3	661.8	371.5	2.746
CHILE: 1960							
Total	3,634.5	2,957.8	676.7	3,776.6	3,067.1	709.5	1.048
0-14	1,491.7	1,102.4	389.3	1,488.0	1,105.6	382.4	.982
15-49	1,685.1	1,497.7	187.4	1,781.6	1,562.6	219.0	1.169
50-64	321.3	261.7	59.6	340.9	281.2	59.7	1.002
65+	136.4	96.0	40.4	166.1	117.6	48.5	1.198

COSTA RICA: 1963							
Total	679.2	554.6	124.6	676.5	553.8	122.7	.985
0-14	332.3	254.2	78.1	324.5	249.3	75.2	.963
15-49	281.6	247.8	33.8	287.1	250.9	36.2	1.071
50-64	44.5	37.1	7.4	44.4	38.0	6.4	.874
65+	20.8	15.5	5.3	20.5	15.5	5.0	.929
EL SALVADOR: 1961							
Total	1,271.7	879.6	392.1	1,307.7	889.0	418.7	1.068
0-14	605.2	371.4	233.8	597.5	356.8	240.7	1.029
15-49	543.1	427.2	115.9	578.8	446.5	132.3	1.141
50-64	86.4	60.4	26.0	90.1	63.2	26.9	1.035
65+	37.0	20.6	16.4	41.3	22.6	18.7	1.144
GUATEMALA: 1964							
Total	2,135.7	1,466.3	669.4	2,145.1	1,451.0	694.1	1.037
0-14	1,006.4	600.5	405.9	996.9	591.6	405.3	.999
15-49	931.2	741.2	190.0	951.6	732.2	219.4	1.155
50-64	140.9	95.2	45.7	139.9	96.7	43.2	.946
65+	57.2	29.3	27.9	56.7	30.5	26.2	.941

Table A-V-3 (continued)

	Populations (thousands)						
	Male			Female			Ratio of Female to Male Difference (6)÷(3)
	Actual	Hypothetical "A"	Difference (1)-(2)	Actual	Hypothetical "A"	Difference (4)-(5)	
Age Group	(1)	(2)	(3)	(4)	(5)	(6)	(7)
			HONDURAS: 1961				
Total	937.4	778.1	159.3	944.0	783.0	161.0	1.010
0-14	456.0	356.9	99.1	445.7	349.1	96.6	.975
15-49	401.3	356.6	44.7	415.0	365.9	49.1	1.099
50-64	58.2	48.2	10.0	58.9	49.5	9.4	.942
65+	21.9	16.3	5.6	24.4	18.6	5.8	1.046
			MEXICO: 1960				
Total	17,812.7	13,915.3	3,897.4	17,880.4	14,025.2	3,855.2	.989
0-14	8,332.8	5,945.0	2,387.8	8,038.5	5,761.1	2,277.4	.954
15-49	7,715.7	6,597.3	1,118.4	8,004.2	6,830.8	1,173.4	1.049
50-64	1,222.8	997.5	225.3	1,259.4	1,025.1	234.3	1.040
65+	541.4	375.5	165.9	578.3	408.2	170.1	1.025
			NICARAGUA: 1963				
Total	756.4	589.8	166.6	775.8	605.6	170.2	1.021
0-14	372.4	269.6	102.8	364.2	263.9	100.3	.976
15-49	318.9	271.1	47.8	339.0	286.6	52.4	1.095
50-64	45.1	35.3	9.8	48.3	38.3	10.0	1.019
65+	20.0	13.8	6.2	24.3	16.8	7.5	1.214

			PANAMA: 1960				
Total	515.1	405.2	109.9	496.5	386.1	110.4	1.005
0-14	220.5	156.4	64.1	215.2	152.6	62.6	.975
15-49	236.4	205.1	31.3	227.0	192.4	34.6	1.107
50-64	39.6	31.5	8.1	36.2	29.1	7.1	.882
65+	18.6	12.2	6.4	18.1	12.0	6.1	.951
			PARAGUAY: 1962				
Total	893.3	722.8	170.5	910.5	737.7	172.8	1.014
0-14	412.1	308.7	103.4	401.4	302.8	98.6	.954
15-49	383.9	338.7	45.2	403.8	352.0	51.8	1.147
50-64	64.5	52.8	11.7	67.7	56.7	11.0	.933
65+	32.8	22.6	10.2	37.6	26.2	11.4	1.121
			VENEZUELA: 1961				
Total	3,865.9	2,797.6	1,068.3	3,743.3	2,694.1	1,049.2	.982
0-14	1,800.7	1,140.9	659.8	1,747.7	1,114.5	633.2	.960
15-49	1,727.2	1,420.4	306.8	1,636.7	1,325.9	310.8	1.013
50-64	254.8	187.1	67.7	250.2	188.6	61.6	.910
65+	83.2	49.2	34.0	108.7	65.2	43.5	1.280

Chapter VI

CONSEQUENCES OF THE MORTALITY DECLINE

Two important effects of the mortality decline in Latin America have been shown: the acceleration of population growth, and the change in the age structure of the population toward a younger configuration. Both effects apparently handicap the efforts of Latin American countries to "improve," at least when their well-being is measured in terms of economic development.

A large body of literature deals with the effect of population growth on economic development. In general, most authors seem to agree that a high population growth rate obstructs economic development of a country, although a few dissenters insist that this is not the case.[1] However, it seems reasonable to assert that when a population expands rapidly over a period of time, substantial economic growth is required to maintain a constant or increasing per capita income, and that such growth cannot be maintained over a long period. In those cases where this tremendous economic advance has been achieved, it is probable that the social conditions would have been better with a slower population growth. A detailed discussion of this complex subject lies outside the scope of this study; however, the impact of changing age structure on an economy is central to it. Let us turn then to an examination of the effects of changing age structure on specific economic indices: dependency ratios, labor force participation, and educational costs.

---

[1]See, for instance: A. Coale and E. Hoover, Population Growth and Economic Development in Low Income Countries (Princeton: Princeton University Press, 1958); Simon Kuznets, et al., eds., Economic Growth: Brazil, India and Japan (Durham, N.C.: Duke University Press, 1955); G. Loyo, Poblacion y Desarrollo Economico (Mexico: Tipografica Londres, 1963); Gallo J. Hubner, El Mito de la Explosion Demografica: La Auto Regulacion Natural de las Poblaciones (Buenos Aires: Joaquin Almendros Press, 1968); several articles in United Nations, Migration, Urbanization and Economic Development, Vol. IV of World Population Conference, 1965 (New York, 1967); Paul Demeny, "Investment Allocation and Population Growth," Demography, 2 (1965): 203-232; Simon Kuznets, "Population and Economic Growth," Proceedings of the American Philosophical Society, III, 3 (June 22, 1967): 170-193; Richard Easterlin, "Effects of Population Growth on the Economic Development of Developing Countries," The Annals, 369 (January 1967): 98-108.

Consequences of Age Structure Changes

Dependency Ratios. The change in the age structure in Latin American countries resulting from mortality decline has increased the number of persons in the economically non-active ages (0-14 and 65+) more than the number in the productive ages (15 to 64). As a consequence, the dependency ratios--the ratios of the populations in non-active ages to those in productive ages--have tended to increase. The difference between the dependency ratios of the actual populations and those of the hypothetical "A" populations--derived when mortality is held constant at the level of the 1930's--shows to what degree the increase in the ratios was due to mortality decline (see Table VI-1). The increase in the ratios averaged .12--from .77 to .89--among the eleven countries (see Chapter V, Table V-7).

Table VI-1

DEPENDENCY RATIOS OF ACTUAL AND HYPOTHETICAL "A" POPULATIONS IN ELEVEN LATIN AMERICAN COUNTRIES: 1960's

	Dependency Ratios			
	$\frac{N_{0-14} + N_{65+}}{N_{15-64}}$		$\frac{N_{0-19} + N_{65+}}{N_{20-64}}$	
Country	Actual	Hypothetical "A"	Actual	Hypothetical "A"
Brazil	.89	.79	1.34	1.21
Chile	.79	.67	1.18	1.02
Costa Rica	1.06	.93	1.60	1.41
El Salvador	.99	.77	1.48	1.17
Guatemala	.98	.75	1.47	1.15
Honduras	1.02	.90	1.54	1.39
Mexico	.96	.81	1.45	1.24
Nicaragua	1.04	.89	1.58	1.37
Panama	.88	.73	1.32	1.11
Paraguay	.96	.83	1.46	1.27
Venezuela				
Total	.97	.76	1.44	1.15
Native[a]	1.07	.84	1.61	1.28
Average[b]	.89	.77	1.35	1.19

[a] See p. 139 below.

[b] The average pertains to the population of the eleven countries combined.

Source: Chapter V, Table V-1, and Appendix V, Table A-V-1.

The change in the dependency ratios resulted principally from an increase in young dependents, who benefitted most from mortality decline. Of the increase of .12 persons in non-active ages per person in active ages, .11 was due to more people under age 15, and only .01 to more 65 and over.

But the dependency ratio as defined above does not give us much information about the average number of people who depend on each worker. This can be obtained by taking the ratio of the total non-active population to the working population. The resulting dependent-active ratio shows a trend similar to that of the dependency ratio, which, if other conditions remain the same, increases with mortality decline. By using the same age-specific participation rates, the total active population can also be found for the hypothetical "A" populations, and the ratio of dependent to active persons for both actual and hypothetical populations can be compared (see Table VI-2). Such a comparison reveals that if the age-specific participation rates had remained constant since the 1930's and only mortality had affected the age structure, the dependent-active ratios in the Latin American countries would have increased by .23 non-active person per active person.

Labor Force Participation. The effect of the changing age structure on labor force participation is reflected in the total labor force participation rate. This rate--the number of economically active people per hundred population--would be expected to decline in Latin America because of the increase of people in non-economically active ages due to the mortality decline (see Table VI-3). However, the total labor force participation for both sexes seems to have remained constant rather than fallen. Before discussing the details of labor force participation in those Latin American countries with more or less reliable data, some general remarks on labor force participation rates in developing countries seem appropriate.

Underdeveloped countries have a higher age-specific labor force participation rate in ages under 15 than do developed countries, because the better economic situation of the latter allows compulsory school attendance for all children up to adolescence. This keeps the younger population out of the labor force. Developing countries, in which school attendance is still rather low, are presently attempting to impose compulsory education, with the result that labor force participation of young ages tends to decline.[2] Thus it is to be expected that labor force

---

[2] The educational variable is probably not the only reason for this declining trend. Improvements in the economic situation of families have also played a role in increasing participation in

Table VI-2

RATIO OF NON-ACTIVE TO ACTIVE PEOPLE IN ACTUAL AND HYPOTHETICAL "A" POPULATIONS, SELECTED LATIN AMERICAN COUNTRIES, BOTH SEXES: 1960's

	Total		Male		Female	
Country	Actual	Hypothetical "A"	Actual	Hypothetical "A"	Actual	Hypothetical "A"
Chile	2.10	1.90	.96	.83	6.08	5.63
Costa Rica	2.41	2.21	1.04	.92	9.43	8.84
El Salvador	2.20	1.90	.93	.75	8.01	7.16
Honduras	2.31	2.15	.89	.80	11.94	11.30
Mexico	2.15	1.95	.91	.78	7.85	7.36
Nicaragua	2.21	2.01	.98	.86	7.06	6.61
Panama	2.00	1.77	.94	.80	5.90	5.40
Venezuela	2.23	1.91	1.02	.82	7.50	6.66
Average[a]	2.20	1.97	.96	.82	7.97	7.36

[a]Average is non-weighted. Actual age-specific activity rules were applied to the projected populations (Chapter V, Appendix V, Table A-V-1). Age-specific activity rates are from United Nations, Demographic Yearbook 1964 (New York, 1965), Table 8.

Source: See note a above.

Table VI-3

TOTAL ACTIVITY RATES OF ACTUAL AND HYPOTHETICAL "A" POPULATIONS IN SELECTED LATIN AMERICAN COUNTRIES: 1960's

(percentages)

		Total		Male		Female	
Country	Year	Actual	Hypothetical "A"	Actual	Hypothetical "A"	Actual	Hypothetical "A"
Chile	1960	32.3	34.5	51.1	54.7	14.1	15.1
Costa Rica	1963	29.4	31.1	49.0	52.0	9.6	10.2
El Salvador	1961	31.2	34.5	51.9	57.0	11.1	12.2
Honduras	1961	30.2	31.7	52.8	55.5	7.7	8.1
Mexico	1960	31.8	33.9	52.3	56.1	11.3	12.0
Nicaragua	1963	31.2	33.2	50.4	53.8	12.4	13.1
Panama	1960	33.3	36.1	51.5	55.6	14.5	15.6
Venezuela	1961	30.9	34.4	49.5	54.9	11.8	13.1
Average[a]		31.3	33.7	51.1	55.0	11.6	12.3

[a]Average is non-weighted. Total activity rates are defined as the ratio of active population to total population. Rates for the projected population were obtained by applying the actual age-specific activity rates to the projected populations of Chapter V, Appendix V, Table A-V-1. Actual age-specific activity rates are from United Nations, Demographic Yearbook 1964 (New York, 1965), Table 8.

Source: See note a above.

participation in developing countries will not increase for the young ages of either sex.

It should be remembered that the age-specific labor force participation rates of adult males in these countries are at levels close to the maximum possible, and that those of old ages tend to decline.[3] Therefore, we would expect that male age-specific labor force participation rates for developing Latin American countries have probably not increased since the 1930's. As a consequence, because of the change in the age structure due to the mortality decline, a reduction in the total male participation rates is likely.[4]

The labor force participation rates for some Latin American countries can be seen in Table VI-4. As expected, the rates for males have tended to decline, except in Venezuela. This country experienced significant immigration during 1950-1960, and most of the immigrants are in the economically active ages. Hence, for a population of natives and foreigners together, the total activity rate for males has not declined. However, the rate for the native male population has fallen significantly.[5]

---

education. See United Nations, Methods of Analyzing Census Data on Economic Activities of the Population: Population Studies, No. 43 (New York, 1968); Juan C. Elizaga, Poblacion Economicamente Activa (Santiago, Chile: Centro Latinoamericano de Demografia, 1964).

[3]The activity rates of old ages in the agricultural sector are greater than in other sectors. Therefore, if there is a shift of male labor from agriculture to other sectors--a concomitant of economic development--a reduction in labor force participation of old ages must be expected (see United Nations, Human Resources of Central America, Panama and Mexico). The possibility also exists that the number of retired persons in old ages will increase.

[4]The census data dealing with economically active populations present problems of accuracy and comparability. The census definition of economically active persons has not remained consistent over time. When it has, the understanding and subjective interpretation of enumerators have changed.

[5]Neither the ratios for the total population nor for the native population are free of biases. They derive, in the first case, from foreigners, and in the second, from the children of foreigners born in Venezuela.

Table VI-4

CENSUS TOTAL ACTIVITY RATES IN SELECTED LATIN AMERICAN COUNTRIES: 1930-1960

(percentages)

Country	Sex	Year			
		1930	1940	1950	1960[a]
Chile	Total		34.7	36.3[b]	32.3
	Male		52.9	55.5	51.2
	Female		16.7	17.8	14.2
El Salvador	Total			35.2	32.1[c]
	Male			59.3	53.4
	Female			11.6	11.5
Mexico	Total	32.3	29.8	32.1	32.4
	Male	61.3	56.0	56.3	52.8
	Female	4.4	4.3	8.6	11.6
Nicaragua	Total			31.2	31.6[d]
	Male			54.5	50.0
	Female			8.6	12.5
Panama	Total		36.7	35.1	33.3
	Male		59.1	55.3	51.1
	Female		13.0	14.2	14.5
Venezuela	Total		32.2[e]	31.8	32.0[c]
	Male		50.4	51.5	51.2
	Female		14.4	11.5	12.1
Venezuela (Native population only)	Total		31.9[e]	27.2	23.4[c]
	Male		50.0	44.2	37.3
	Female		14.3	10.3	9.5

[a]The rates for the 1960's differ from those of Table VI-3 because rates of this table are derived from populations given in the censuses. Rates of Table VI-3 were also calculated from census populations, but after correction for underenumeration in ages under 10 and after smoothing the age structure.

[b]1952 [c]1961 [d]1963 [e]1941

Source: See note a above.

In contrast to the decline of male participation, the total activity rate for both sexes combined remained almost constant between the last two census dates. This was because of the increase in female participation rates. We now face an interesting question. Why have female labor participation rates increased in Latin America? Do women want to work, or must they work in order to maintain family income levels (or, more technically, the same actual average dependent-active ratio)? In other words, is the female rate change from 1950 to 1960 a consequence of changing attitudes toward work because of changing aspirations, or is it due to the necessity of contributions to the family income? Unfortunately, census data do not enable us to answer these questions; a survey would be required. Nevertheless, some census material seems to support the view that some females are working because they have to, rather than because they want to. These data show that a very high proportion of economically active females in Latin America are still in domestic service. In the following table, the domestic service rate is compared to that for other sectors for those countries with the necessary census information:

Female Labor Participation Rates[a]

(per thousand)

Country	Year	Total	Domestic Services	Other Occupations
Costa Rica	1950	104.3	40.0	64.3
	1963	96.5	22.5	74.0
Mexico	1960	116.1	27.9	88.3
Panama	1960	145.2	39.7	105.5
Venezuela	1950	103.1	31.8	71.3
	1961	95.4	24.4	71.0

[a]The rates are defined as the total active population divided by the total female population in all ages.

It is reasonable to assume that the presence of most women in domestic services is contrary to their wishes. It is known that when countries advance economically, this sector of the female labor force almost disappears, as women shift from domestic services to other industry sectors.[6]

At present there is almost no information about the fertility of females working in domestic services in Latin America. The only available survey, conducted in Lima, Peru, concluded that married females in the labor force have as many children as those outside the labor force.[7] Since childhood mortality decline has been to a great extent independent of the economic situation, more children than ever are surviving in poor and less educated families. As a consequence, and as the data from the Lima survey suggest, uneducated mothers with several children have possibly been forced into domestic services because of economic necessity. This is merely an assumption which unfortunately at the present time cannot be proved with the information available.

Educational Costs. Another consequence of the changing age structure in the population resulting from mortality decline

---

[6]For example, the average of the rates of women's work-participation in private domestic service and all other occupations given by Collver and Langlois for two different groups of countries are:

Work-Participation Rates in the 1950's[a]

Country Group	Total	Private Domestic Service	All Occupations Excluding Private Domestic Service
United States, Canada, England and Wales, Belgium, Switzerland and France	39.6	3.7	35.9
Venezuela, Brazil, Paraguay, El Salvador, Nicaragua	35.2	13.4	21.8

[a]The work-participation rate is the ratio of the labor force to the population aged 15-64, as defined on page 369 of the source article.

Source: Calculated from Andrew Collver and Eleanor Langlois, "The Female Labor Force in Metropolitan Areas: An International Comparison," Economic Development and Cultural Change, X, No. 4 (July, 1962): 367-385, Table 1.

[7]Mayone Stycos, Human Fertility in Latin America (Ithaca: Cornell University Press, 1968), pp. 236-249.

has been an increase in the cost of education per productive individual. The education of youth is paid for through the tax and budgetary systems by the labor force. With conditions of attendance and cost per student constant and no change in labor force participation rates, the cost of education per worker has increased because of the mortality decline. The average cost of education per worker for the eleven Latin American countries analyzed herein is presumed to have increased, due to the mortality decline since the 1930's, around 13 percent, holding economic and educational variables constant.[8] This increase would have been registered if only mortality had changed. The actual rise has probably been greater than 13 percent, since school attendance rates have grown during this period, as is indicated by an increased proportion of young literates in the censuses. The growing proportion of literates in the population 15 years old and over for countries with information for the 1950's and the 1960's is indicated in the following table:

Percent of Population 15 Years Old and Over
Who are Literate

Country	1950's	1960's
Brazil	49.3	60.5
Chile	79.8	83.6
Costa Rica	79.4	84.4
El Salvador	38.4	49.0
Guatemala	29.4	37.9
Honduras	35.2	47.3
Mexico	55.9	62.2
Nicaragua	38.4	49.8
Panama	69.9	76.6
Venezuela	51.0	63.3

Source: Pan American Union, Inter-American Statistical Institute, America en Cifras 1965, Situacion Cultural: Educacion y otros Aspectos Culturales (Washington, D.C., 1967).

[8] For the eleven countries combined, the ratios of the population under age 15 to workers in the actual and hypothetical "A" populations (using the same age-specific participation rates) were 1.394 and 1.216 respectively. The former ratio is 14.6 percent higher than the latter.

It should be kept in mind that the cost of education per worker is being considered, not the indirect benefit that each country

Conclusions

The mortality decline in Latin America has caused a sharp increase in total population growth and a proportionately younger population, both of which have slowed the economic development of countries in this area. The impact of these changes has been exacerbated by the continued high fertility rates in the region. During the 30-year period of exceptional mortality control, fertility has been left virtually unaffected; its reduction could have counteracted the change in the age structure due to mortality decline. In the next chapters we shall analyze the fertility variable, but here we should note the effect of the altered age structure (resulting from drastic mortality decline) on the crude birth rate. The mortality decline increased the population in all ages, but to varying degrees. The proportion of females in the fertile ages from 15 to 49 who were alive due to the mortality decline was 13.3 percent of the enumerated population in the same ages. The proportion for the rest of the population (including males--see Chapter V) was 21.7 percent. In other words, the reduction of mortality has tended, in relative terms, to _reduce_ the number of potential "children producers." Therefore, the failure of actual crude birth rates to decline in most Latin American countries shows that certain factors tended to _increase_ fertility. The question of whether mortality decline was one of these factors will be considered in the next chapter.

---

receives from a declining mortality among already educated persons. In other words, we are not considering the losses of educational investments due to mortality conditions. However, a model using the stable population theory, and taking into account the losses of all investments in education due to the annual deaths of students up to age 24 and the annual cost of education per worker, shows that the decline of mortality registered in Latin American countries has produced an increase in the cost of education greater than the decline of losses of investments in education per worker. In other words, because of the change in the age structure due to mortality decline, the increase in the cost of education for each worker is greater than the decrease of investment lost due to the deaths of students. In the model, two stable populations differing only in the level of mortality are compared for each country. All the attendance rates of students, activity rates of the population, age-specific fertility rates, and annual student costs per age are held constant.

P A R T IV

THE RESPONSE OF FERTILITY

Chapter VII

THE EFFECT OF RAPID MORTALITY DECLINE ON LATIN AMERICAN FERTILITY

Never before in history has a region of the world shown as sharp a contrast between birth and death rates as Latin America now shows (see Tables VII-1 and VII-2). This unprecedented contrast of rates is only one of the consequences of the mortality decline, which has also affected fertility in two apparently opposing ways.[1] Since mortality decline affects all ages, the average life span of couples throughout the reproductive period has been extended, and an increase of age-specific fertility rates has been registered. At the same time, however, the change of the population age structure caused by the mortality decline has tended to reduce the crude birth rates. In this chapter we shall first analyze how mortality has affected crude birth rates, and then how it has influenced age-specific fertility rates.

The Effect of the Mortality Decline on the Crude Birth Rate

The mortality decline in Latin America, which has caused the age structure of the population to shift toward the younger ages, has meant that proportionately smaller numbers of people are in the reproductive ages. This in turn has influenced the crude birth rates. As the reader will remember, the proportion of females between the ages of 15 and 49 "saved" from death because of the mortality decline represented about 13.3 percent of the enumerated population between these ages in the 1960's, while in the rest of the population (both sexes) the percentage of "saved" people was around 21.7. As a consequence, since the

---

[1]The indices generally used in measuring fertility are: (1) the crude birth rate, which takes account of the whole population; (2) the age-specific fertility rates of all females, which include all women in the fertile ages--even those not exposed to the risk of conception; and (3) the age-specific fertility rates of married females. The three indices are very closely related, and their trends are usually similar, although sometimes exceptions can be observed. The crude birth rate is affected primarily by the age structures of both sexes, while the age-specific fertility rate of females depends mainly on the marital age distribution of the population.

Table VII-1

ESTIMATED CRUDE DEATH RATES IN ELEVEN LATIN AMERICAN COUNTRIES: 1930-1960[a]

(per thousand)

	Five-Year Periods					
Country	1930-34	1935-39	1940-44	1945-49	1950-54	1955-59
Brazil	32.5	30.2	27.4	23.9	19.9	15.0
Chile	30.7	29.0	25.9	21.0	14.7	13.3
Costa Rica	23.5	20.2	17.2	14.2	11.7	9.7
El Salvador	37.0	30.9	25.5	20.9	17.3	14.1
Guatemala	41.4	35.7	29.2	22.8	18.5	16.4
Honduras	31.8	29.3	26.7	23.7	20.4	16.0
Mexico	29.0	26.4	23.4	19.9	16.1	12.9
Nicaragua	38.5	34.9	31.2	27.1	22.9	18.1
Panama	28.3	24.8	21.7	18.5	15.2	11.5
Paraguay	31.5	28.8	25.9	22.4	18.7	15.0
Venezuela	32.9	28.3	21.8	16.1	11.7	8.9
Average	32.5	29.0	25.1	21.0	17.0	13.7

[a]These rates were estimated in this study during the rejuvenation of the populations.

Table VII-2

CRUDE BIRTH RATES IN ELEVEN LATIN AMERICAN COUNTRIES: 1930-1960

(per thousand)

Country	Five-Year Periods					
	1930-34	1935-39	1940-44	1945-49	1950-54	1955-59
Brazil[a]	44.1	44.9	46.0	46.4	46.8	44.0
Chile[b]	40.2	38.4	38.3	37.0	37.0	37.6
Costa Rica[b]	44.6	43.3	42.8	42.7	45.0	45.3
El Salvador[b]	46.5	45.4	45.2	44.8	47.9	47.9
Guatemala[b]	46.2	44.2	45.2	49.1	50.9	49.0
Honduras[b]	42.0	41.9	43.8	44.5	46.0	46.0
Mexico[b]	44.1	43.5	43.8	44.5	45.0	45.8
Nicaragua[a]	42.9	45.7	48.7	50.7	52.9	50.6
Panama[b]	37.4	37.8	39.5	38.3	38.5	40.5
Paraguay[a]	38.8	41.3	44.7	45.8	46.2	43.9
Venezuela[b]	39.9	40.2	41.5	43.6	44.2	44.3
Average[c]	42.4	42.4	43.6	44.3	45.5	45.0

[a]Estimated in this study by rejuvenation process.

[b]From Collver, Birth Rates, Table 5.

[c]The average is non-weighted.

number of potential mothers has been reduced in relation to the total population because of the mortality decline, we would expect that under conditions of no change in the age-specific fertility rates, the crude birth rates would decline.

Contrary to expectation, however, the official crude birth rates for most Latin American countries have increased (see Table VII-3). It is possible that a considerable part of the rate increase is due to improved reporting and registration of births; certainly the degree of completeness of the registers has not been particularly high.[2] Consequently, estimated crude birth rates for these countries give a more accurate picture than official data. Collver's estimates are given in Table VII-2, and they show that all countries have had rising crude birth rates from the 1930's to the 1960's except Chile. The average estimated birth rate for all countries rose from a level of 42.4 in the 1930's to 45.0 per thousand in the 1960's.

Let us now determine the expected crude birth rate trend under conditions of changing mortality and constant age-specific fertility rates. A standardization will be made in order to detect the change in the crude birth rate caused by the mortality decline. The same age-specific fertility rates will be applied to the actual and hypothetical "A" populations for each country in the 1960's.[3] (The hypothetical "A" populations are those of

---

[2]For estimates of completeness, see Collver, Birth Rates, Table 6. Also Zulma Camisa, "Assessment of Registration and Census Data on Fertility," Milbank Memorial Fund Quarterly, XLVI, No. 3 (July 1968): 19, Table J.

[3]Age-specific fertility rates are usually derived from birth registers. The official age-specific fertility rates for the Latin American countries have not been used in this study because the birth registers in most of them still contain inaccuracies, the most common being late registrations. Chile provides a good example. Official birth data are usually considered to be complete (see United Nations, Demographic Yearbook 1965). However, the Bulletin No. 12, Direccion de Estadistica, Dic. 1962, page 341, gives the number of registered births in Chile during the year by the age of the registered human being. The registrants are divided into those under age two and those two and over. From 1951 to 1960, the annual average of registered births "at two and over years old" was 15 percent of the total registered (a maximum of 22.2 percent in 1954 and a minimum of 9.5 in 1959). The same statistical office also publishes Demografia, which contains an estimate of the births occurring each year, considered to be the official figure. The estimation is made as follows:

Table VII-3

OFFICIAL CRUDE BIRTH RATES IN SELECTED LATIN AMERICAN COUNTRIES: 1930 TO 1960

(per thousand)

Country	Five-Year Periods						
	1930-34	1935-39	1940-44	1945-49	1950-54	1955-59	1960[a]
Chile	40.5	36.6	36.4	35.7	33.8	35.8	35.5
Costa Rica	45.7	45.0	44.9	45.1	48.7	48.8	45.0
El Salvador	43.3	42.7	43.3	44.4	48.4	47.4	48.0
Guatemala	51.6	47.7	47.2	50.6	51.4	49.1	47.0
Honduras	33.5	35.6	36.7	38.6	40.8	42.4	48.5
Mexico	44.5	43.5	44.2	44.4	44.9	45.9	44.5
Nicaragua	35.9	40.3	38.8	40.2	42.1	47.5	48.5
Panama	36.5	36.4	37.5	36.0	37.5	39.8	41.5
Paraguay	31.6	31.6	37.2	43.0	46.6	43.5	43.5
Venezuela	28.2	32.7	35.7	38.5	43.7	44.1	47.0
Average[b]	39.1	39.2	40.2	41.6	43.8	44.4	44.9

[a] The levels of this column are the mean point of the interval level given by the United Nations.

[b] Average is non-weighted.

Source: United Nations, Demographic Yearbook 1959, 1963, and 1966 (New York: 1959, 1964, and 1967), Tables 9, 19, and 7 respectively. For Chile 1960, Chile, Direccion de Estadistica y Censo, Demografia Año 1962, p. 33.

Chapter V, which differ from the actual only in that mortality conditions were held constant at 1930's levels in their calculation.) The age-specific fertility rates for each country which are applied to both populations are given in Table VII-4. The product of these rates by the populations of each country gives the total number of births, and the total births divided by the total populations gives the crude birth rates. The difference between the two crude birth rates of the actual and hypothetical "A" populations represents the effect of mortality decline on the crude birth rate. As Table VII-5 shows, actual crude birth rates in all countries were lower than those that would have been registered if mortality had not changed since the 1930's. The average crude birth rate for the hypothetical "A" populations with constant mortality is 50.1 per thousand; the average crude birth rate for the actual populations is 45.5. For individual countries, a decline in birth rate ranging from approximately 7 to 14 percent from 1930 to 1960 would be expected, given no change in age-specific fertility rates for females. Since in fact crude birth rates did not decline (see Table VII-2 and VII-3), it is clear that somehow age-specific fertility rates increased. The exception is Chile, where the actual crude birth rate has been falling. This country will be analyzed separately later; first it is necessary to examine precisely how mortality has affected age-specific fertility rates.

> "From 1938 to 1951, live births are calculated by increasing the number of persons registered at age under two years old by 9.5 percent; from 1952 to the present, the estimate of actual births is made by increasing by 5 percent the number of live births occurring during each year but registered from January 1 to March 31 of the next year." (Chile, Direccion de Estadistica y Censos, Demografia 1962 [Santiago, Chile], p. 32n.)

Unfortunately, the basis for the 5 and 9.5 percent increases is not explained.

In most of the other countries the situation is worse: officials do not attempt any correction. Thus, rather than use the official age-specific fertility rates for each country, an estimation of the total births (or birth rates) and the official proportional distribution of births by mothers' ages were used to calculate the age-specific fertility rates. The number of births in Chile, Costa Rica, Mexico, and Venezuela at the last census date were taken from previous estimates made by the author (Arriaga, New Life Tables). The estimates of the birth rates previously used in this chapter were applied for the rest of the countries.

Estimates of births or birth rates do not affect the analyses and results of this study, the purpose of which is to study the trends rather than the levels of fertility.

Table VII-4

ACTUAL AGE-SPECIFIC FERTILITY RATES IN ELEVEN LATIN AMERICAN COUNTRIES: 1960's

Country	Gross Reproduction Rate	Age Groups						
		15-19	20-24	25-29	30-34	35-39	40-44	45-49
Brazil	2.99	.09655	.28217	.30087	.24297	.19819	.08502	.01890
Chile	2.48	.07956	.21642	.25278	.22941	.16092	.06436	.01443
Costa Rica	3.52	.11166	.33802	.35579	.30246	.22709	.09317	.01595
El Salvador	3.30	.13652	.33494	.33655	.25922	.19398	.06958	.02034
Guatemala	3.40	.15909	.32350	.32420	.27207	.20852	.08199	.02523
Honduras	3.49	.14729	.32045	.34753	.28764	.21633	.08954	.02391
Mexico	3.17	.10241	.29932	.31915	.25775	.21021	.09032	.01991
Nicaragua	3.45	.14542	.36867	.37674	.24806	.19116	.06567	.02042
Panama	2.68	.14831	.30380	.27672	.19170	.12944	.04183	.00845
Paraguay	3.15	.10433	.29778	.29308	.26593	.21626	.09262	.02268
Venezuela	3.31	.13407	.33742	.34403	.26458	.19402	.06468	.01960
Average[a]	3.18	.12411	.31114	.32068	.25656	.19510	.07618	.01907

[a] Average is non-weighted.

Source: Calculated from distribution of birth by age of mother (from United Nations, Demographic Yearbook 1965, Table 13), estimates of crude birth rates (from Table VII-2), and country's population (from Appendix V, Table A-V-1). Also see footnote 3 above. Rates for Brazil are those of Mexico reduced proportionately to the relative difference of the crude birth rates for these two countries (see Table VII-2).

Table VII-5

CRUDE BIRTH RATES FOR ACTUAL AND HYPOTHETICAL "A" POPULATIONS IN ELEVEN LATIN AMERICAN COUNTRIES: 1960's[a]

(per thousand)

	Birth Rates		Differences	
	Actual Population	Hypothetical "A" Population	Absolute (2)-(1)	Percent (3)÷(1)
Country	(1)	(2)	(3)	(4)
Brazil	44.0	47.5	3.5	7.9
Chile	37.1	40.4	3.3	8.8
Costa Rica	47.0	50.5	3.5	7.5
El Salvador	47.9	54.5	6.6	13.8
Guatemala	49.0	56.0	7.0	14.3
Honduras	49.7	53.1	3.4	6.9
Mexico	45.0	49.5	4.5	10.1
Nicaragua	50.6	55.2	4.6	9.1
Panama	40.3	43.8	3.5	8.6
Paraguay	44.0	47.7	3.7	8.4
Venezuela	46.1	52.4	6.3	13.6
Average[b]	45.52	50.05	4.54	9.91

[a]The crude birth rates were calculated by obtaining the total number of births from the age-specific fertility rates of Table VII-4 and the actual and hypothetical "A" populations, Chapter V, Appendix V, Table A-V-1.

[b]Average is non-weighted.

RESPONSE OF FERTILITY

The Effect of the Mortality Decline on Age-Specific Fertility Rates

Falling mortality can affect age-specific fertility rates in one way by modifying the marital distribution of females during the period they are exposed to the "risk" of having children.[4] There is no doubt that a mortality decline such as the one registered in Latin America since the 1930's usually increases the proportion of females living in marital unions. Let us consider why this happens.

The reproductive life of a woman depends not only on her own life, but also on the life of her mate. Therefore, for a thorough fertility analysis, the reproductive union of man and woman should be considered a unit. The "life" of such a unit depends on the joint survival of the woman and man involved. In Latin America, during the period 1930-1960, the survival probability of a couple rose faster than the survival probability of an individual person.[5] As a consequence, the probabilities of survival of married women increased more rapidly than those of single women. (Of course, the probability in general of a woman surviving is greater than that of her surviving as a married woman.) In relative terms, therefore, married women will increase more than women in other civil status categories (if there is no increase in divorces), and hence an increase in the proportion of married females is to be expected when mortality declines.[6]

The number of life-years of a couple as a unit has increased considerably in Latin America since the 1930's. The index ${}_{n}AC_{x,y}^{t,t+i}$ explained in Chapter IV, Appendix IV-1, allows us to calculate this increase--that is, the average rise in the number of years to be lived jointly by a woman age x and a man age y during the next n years due to change in mortality conditions from those of year t to those of year t+i.

---

[4]Arriaga, "Effect of the Decline in Mortality."

[5]This is because of the combined effect of the increase of each factor on the increase of the product. For instance, in Chile the probability of a woman age 25 surviving to age 50 was .6669 in 1930 and .8827 in 1960. If we assume she was married to a man age 30, whose probability of surviving 25 years more was .5987 and .7776 in 1930 and 1960 respectively, the joint probability of the couple surviving 25 years more was .3993 in 1930 and .6864 in 1960.

[6]Arriaga, "Effect of the Decline in Mortality."

Assuming that females 20 years old married or in unions have mates 5 years older (this is very close to the actual marital age differential in Latin America for that age of female), the $_{n}AC^{t,t+i}_{x:y}$ index calculated for the period from the 1930's to the 1960's shows how many years longer couples--where brides and grooms are 20 and 25 years old, respectively--lived on the average in the 1960's because of improved mortality conditions since the 1930's (see Table VII-6). For the eleven Latin American countries combined, females in unions or marriages lived 6.3 years longer on the average under mortality conditions of the 1960's than they lived under conditions of the 1930's. In Chapter IV we saw that the increase in life span for all females aged 20 to 49 was only 3.9 years. By comparing this figure with that for females in unions, it is clear that married couples profited more by the mortality decline than females as a whole.

Therefore, it can be concluded that in those countries where the fertility of married women did not change, the decline of mortality increased the age-specific fertility rates for all females. Indeed, in one case, even though marital fertility fell, the age-specific fertility rates for all females rose because the decline was counteracted by a rise in the proportion of married females resulting from declined mortality.[7] But increased age-specific fertility rates of married females are also to be expected from improved prenatal mother care and better nutritional and female sanitary conditions, allowing women to carry pregnancy to full term.[8]

In fact, age-specific fertility rates rose in all countries considered here, except Chile. Whether the increase in the rates was due only to the growth in the proportion of married women in reproductive ages, or also in part to the rise of age-specific fertility rates for married females--both of which conditions resulted in part from mortality decline--is almost impossible to establish because of lack of information.

The Chilean Case

Chile is the only country of the eleven considered here which shows a decline in birth rates, detected not only in

---

[7] This occurred in Venezuela. See ibid.

[8] Anne Retel-Laurentin, "Influence de certaines maladies sur la fecondite, un exemple africain," Population, 22, No. 5 (Sept.-Oct., 1967): 841-860.

Table VII-6

TEMPORARY 30-YEAR LIFE EXPECTANCIES AND ABSOLUTE CHANGES FOR COUPLES, WOMEN AGE 20 AND MEN AGE 25, IN ELEVEN LATIN AMERICAN COUNTRIES: 1930's TO 1960's

Country	$/30\ e^{1930}_{20:25}$	$/30\ e^{1960}_{20:25}$	$_{30}AC^{30-60}_{20:25}$
Brazil	19.4287	25.6715	6.2428
Chile	20.1540	25.8594	5.7054
Costa Rica	22.5875	27.7233	5.1357
El Salvador	18.3777	25.8437	7.4660
Guatemala	17.1295	24.6023	7.4729
Honduras	19.7108	25.5121	5.8112
Mexico	19.7506	25.5442	5.7936
Nicaragua	18.7901	25.0575	6.2674
Panama	20.5116	26.8868	6.3752
Paraguay	20.3570	25.7490	5.3920
Venezuela	19.3264	26.8608	7.5345
Average[a]	19.6476	25.9373	6.2892

[a] Average is non-weighted.

official data[9] but in estimated figures as well.[10] Chile also appears to have the highest proportion of contraceptive users and the highest abortion rate of the eleven countries.[11] In spite of this, however, an analysis of the data indicates that age-specific fertility rates have not declined; the falling birth rate from 1930 to 1960 occurred mainly because of the impact of mortality decline on the age structure of the population. This conclusion is based on two principal findings: (a) the crude birth rates estimated by Collver show a decline very close to that to be expected from the mortality effect on the age structure (see Collver's figures in Table VI-2 and Table VI-5), and (b) the crude birth rates for 1930 and 1960--41.3 and 37.6 per thousand, respectively--obtained by applying the same age-specific fertility rates to the actual census populations in 1930 and 1960, show a decline which is also close to that in (a).[12]

Examining the situation more closely, we find that the proportion of females living in marriages and consensual unions has risen in all reproductive ages, according to the last two censuses. (There is no information concerning consensual unions in the 1930 or 1940 censuses.)[13] Therefore, if age-specific fertility rates for females have remained almost constant, and if

---

[9] Chile, Direccion de Estadistica y Censo, Demografia 1956 and Demografia 1960.

[10] Collver, Birth Rates.

[11] Studies conducted after 1960 show that the Chilean population has adopted contraceptive methods and abortion. From the number of abortions for certain ages, it must be concluded that such attitudes were quite widely accepted before 1960. See Mario Requena, "Social and Economic Correlates of Induced Abortion in Santiago, Chile," Demography, 2 (1965): 33-49.

[12] Almost the same official crude birth rates are given by country (Table VI-6), Collver (Table VI-2), and Table VI-5.

[13] The percentages of women in marriages and consensual unions to total females was:

Age	1952	1960
15-19	8.71	9.34
20-24	40.51	41.69
25-29	62.51	64.86
30-34	71.65	74.28
35-39	73.91	75.81
40-44	71.46	74.23
45-49	67.16	70.81

the proportion of women in marriages and consensual unions has increased, it seems logical to conclude that age-specific fertility rates for women in marriages and consensual unions have decreased. This decline, as well as the efforts made by the population to reduce the fertility of the total female population, have been counterbalanced by the impact of the mortality decline--at least up to 1960. In the only country where the crude birth rate was actually declining, the decline appears to have been due to the effect of mortality decline on the age structure, and not to the voluntary efforts of women to reduce their fertility. However, if the married females continue reducing their fertility in the future, a decline of the age-specific fertility rates for all women will occur. This is what has been happening in Chile since 1960, judging by the official statistics up to 1967, which give a crude birth rate of 30 per thousand.

Conclusion

In sum, the impact of declining mortality on fertility in Latin American countries has been illusory. The fertility trend has usually been measured in terms of crude birth rates--which for most of the countries have increased slightly or remained constant. This fact has concealed the actual trend of female fertility, which has been an increase in the number of children per female in fertile ages. The only country in which birth rates fell from 1930 to 1960--Chile--experienced the decline because of the effect of mortality decline on the age structure. Although it appears that a decline in the fertility of married females may have begun in Chile, this decline--up to 1960--had not been large enough to counteract the births from the increase of the proportion of married females.

These percentages were calculated from Chile, Servicio Nacional de Estadistica y Censos, *XII Censo General de Poblacion y I de Vivienda, Tomo I, Resumen del Pais* (Santiago, Chile, 1956), p. 134, and Chile, Direccion de Estadistica y Censos, *Poblacion del Pais, Caracteristicas Basicas de la Poblacion (Censo 1960)* (Santiago, Chile, 1964), p. 16.

Chapter VIII

THE LATIN AMERICAN VERSUS THE EUROPEAN MODEL

The failure of fertility to decline in response to the fall of mortality in Latin America indicates a demographic pattern very different from the European historical pattern. We will first analyze the respective mortality-fertility patterns in Europe and Latin America, and then illustrate the differences between them by calculating the Latin American populations as they would have been had they possessed the same fertility level as the European populations at the same mortality level. A comparison of the resulting hypothetical populations for Latin America with the actual populations will show the effect of the different mortality-fertility relationship in Latin America. In order to differentiate them from the hypothetical "A" populations of Chapter V, we will call the projected populations in this chapter hypothetical "B" populations.

The Mortality-Fertility Relationships in Europe and Latin America

Both mortality and fertility have been declining in Europe for a long period of time. The character and causes of this fall have been extensively analyzed by other researchers,[1] who have shown, among other things, that the differences between the levels of mortality and fertility in Europe (measured in terms of crude death and birth rates) have remained within a small range.[2]

---

[1] Jacques Bertillon, La dépopulation de la France (Paris: Librairie Félix Alcan, 1911), pp. 90-137; Kingsley Davis, "The World Demographic Transition," Annals of the American Academy of Political and Social Science, 237 (Jan. 1945): 1-11, and "The Theory of Change and Response in Modern Demographic History," Population Index, 29, No. 4 (Oct. 1963): 345-366; E.F. Penrose, Population Theories and their Application (Food Research Institute, Stanford University, 1934). See also several articles in Clyde V. Kiser and P.K. Whelpton, eds., Social and Psychological Factors Affecting Fertility, Vols. I to V (New York: The Milbank Memorial Fund, 1958).

[2] See especially Kuczynski, The Balance of Births and Deaths, Vols. I and II, and Egon Vielrose, Elements of the National Movement of Population (Pergamon Press, 1965).

This relationship between mortality and fertility seems independent of time and country in Europe. A given mortality level (measured in terms of life expectancy at birth) is generally associated with a certain crude birth rate level, whatever the country and time in history. If a graph of life expectancies and crude birth rates is made, using data from any year (see Figure VIII-1), there is a biunivocal relationship between the two. This relationship can be analytically expressed by fitting a third degree polynomial function to the data,[3] which gives a coefficient of correlation of $R^2 = .915$. The function is

$$1000b = 98.2466 - 2.353774(e_0) + .02306717(e_0)^2 - .0000825387(e_0)^3$$

(VIII-1)

This function has meaning only for levels of life expectancy between 25 and 75. For life expectancy levels of 30 and 55, the estimated crude birth rates are 46.2 and 24.8 respectively.

The relationship between crude birth rates and life expectancies in Latin America is completely different from that in Europe. Graphing the function correlating the values of birth rates and life expectancies shows that for practically any life expectancy the estimated crude birth rate remains at almost the same level. As in the European case, a third degree function was fitted to the data by the least square method; the function obtained is

$$1000.b = 75.5518 - 2.182631(e_0) + .04870268(e_0)^2 - .0003526065(e_0)^3$$

(VIII-2)

and the coefficient of correlation, $R^2 = .05193$. In this case, it seems that both variables are independent and no special correspondence exists between them, although the adjusted third degree polynomial is a good estimate of Latin American birth rates between the life expectancy levels of 25 and 65 (see Figure VIII-2). The polynomial function gives estimated crude birth rates of 44.4 and 44.2 per thousand for the life expectancy levels at birth of 30 and 55 years, respectively. In Europe as well as in Latin America, when mortality was very high (low life expectancy), the birth rate was also high. But there is a great difference in birth rates once mortality declines--24.8 for Europe

[3]The third degree polynomial fit best among first, second, and third degree polynomials and an exponential function.

Figure VIII-1

CRUDE BIRTH RATES AND LIFE EXPECTANCIES AT BIRTH IN EUROPEAN COUNTRIES: HISTORICAL DATA

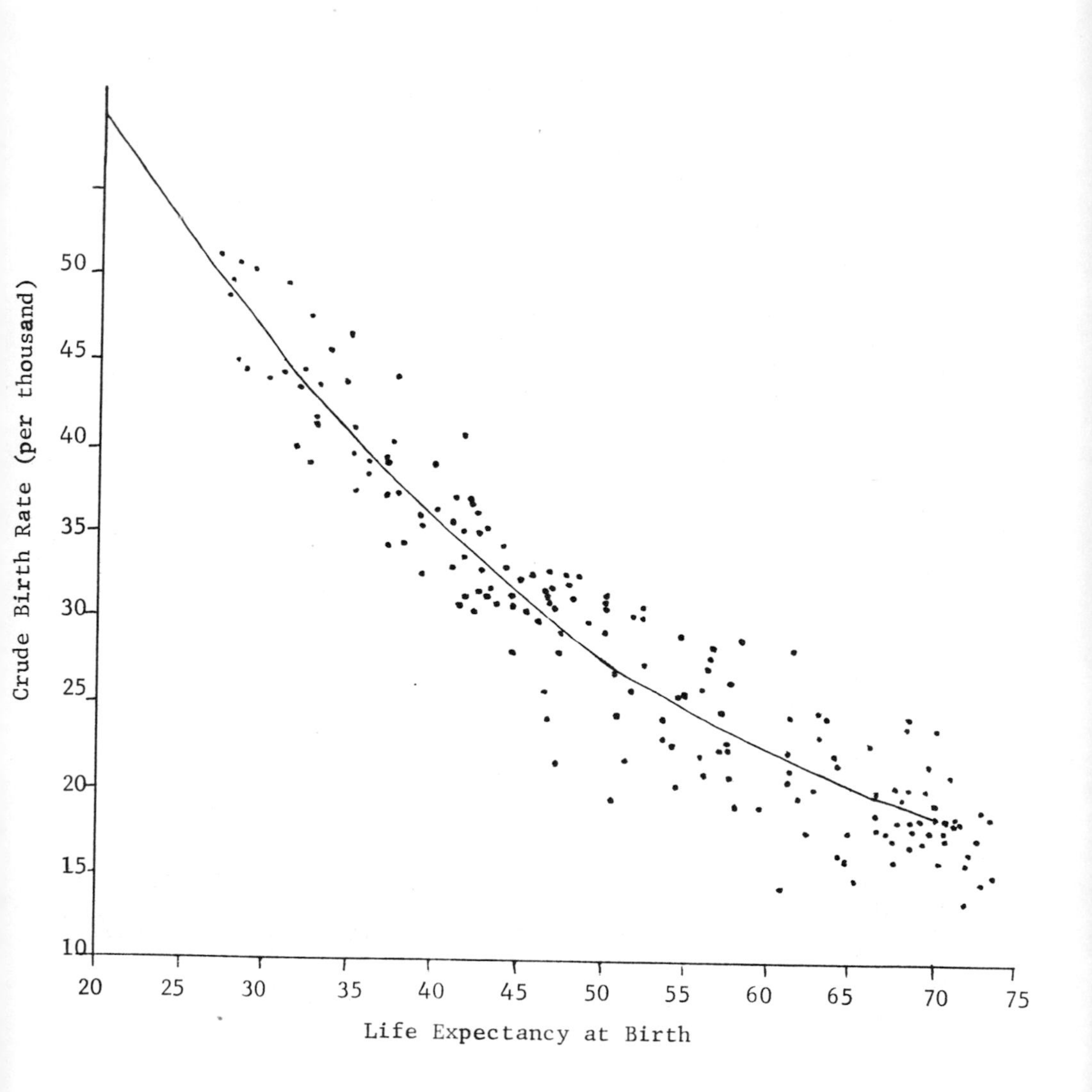

Figure VIII-2

CRUDE BIRTH RATES AND LIFE EXPECTANCIES AT BIRTH IN LATIN AMERICAN COUNTRIES: HISTORICAL DATA

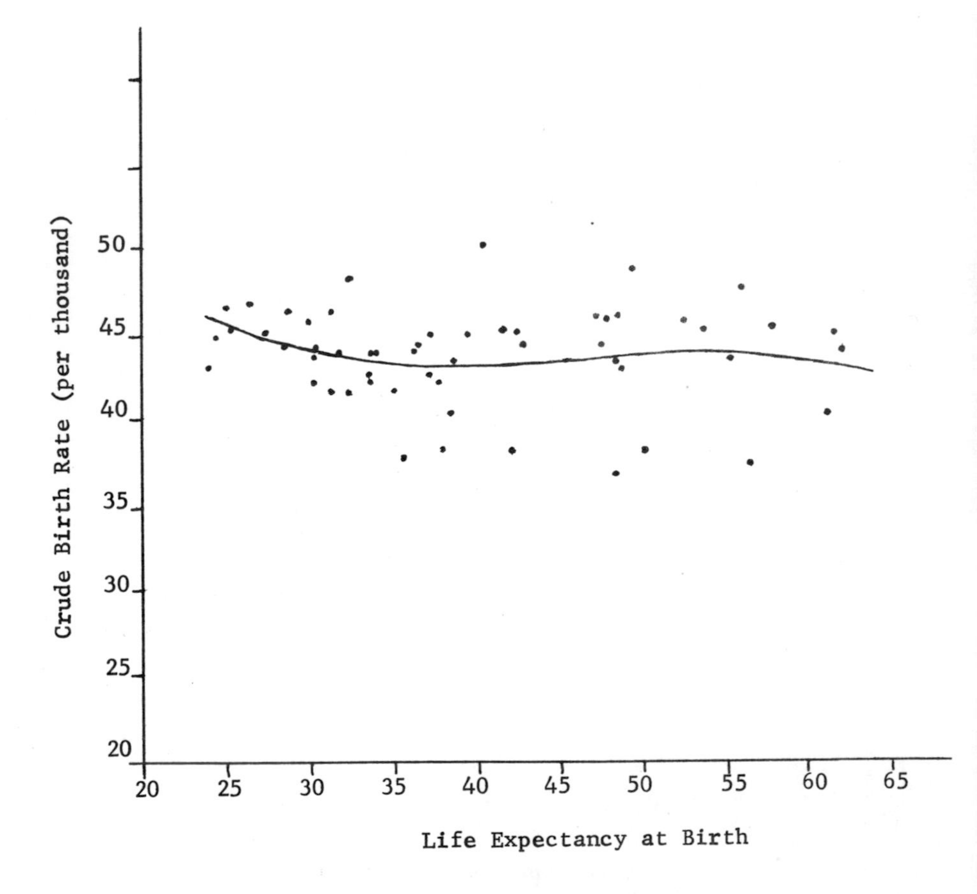

compared to 44.2 for Latin America at a life expectancy level of 55.

The difference in the mortality-fertility patterns of Latin America and Europe raises two questions: what would be the condition of the Latin American populations if they had had the European mortality-fertility relationship, and what would the consequences of such a hypothetical situation have been? To answer these two questions, populations from the 1930's to the 1960's can be projected for Latin American countries on the basis of the European mortality-fertility model, and these hypothetical "B" populations compared with actual Latin American statistics from the period.

Hypothetical "B" Latin American Populations Based on the European Mortality-Fertility Model

The method of projecting these hypothetical populations very closely resembles that used in Chapter V. The difference lies in the assumptions which are made. The fertility levels in Chapter V were the actual ones, and mortality was the variable assumed constant during the projection period; in the present case, the actual (changing) mortality of the period 1930 to 1960 is used, with fertility decreasing. Crude birth rates are obtained with the third degree polynomial function used for the European data (VIII-1), which provides an estimate for any particular date by treating the country's life expectancy level at that date as the independent variable in the equation. As in Chapter V, the projections cover the span from the 1930's to the 1960's, and the base population of the projection is the rejuvenated population of each country. The same survivors ratios used in the rejuvenation process are utilized here,[4] and instead of age-specific fertility rates, crude birth rates are used for the same reasons given earlier. The methodology is exactly the same as in Chapter V, except that the formula used to obtain the total number of births for each of the 5-year periods of the projection is not formula A-V-15 (Chapter V, Appendix V), but is

$$B^{t,t+5} = \frac{b^{t}.N^{t} + b^{t+5}.N_{5+}^{t+5}}{.4 - P_{b}^{t,t+5}.b^{t+5}} \qquad \text{(VIII-3)}$$

where each of the symbols represents exactly the same variable it did in Chapter V.[5] The survivors at ages 0-4 were found

[4] Thus, the difference between the projected and actual populations is due only to the different crude birth rates.

[5] This formula was deduced from formulae A-V-1, A-V-2, A-V-12, and A-V-13 from Chapter V, Appendix V.

as before by using the period masculinity rates at birth and the survivor ratios for births. The crude birth rates used in the projection can be seen in Table VIII-1.

The hypothetical "B" populations in the 1960's will differ from the census enumerations only for ages under 30. Due to the fact that only birth rates have been changed--mortality rates being the actual ones--only the numbers of survivors born since the 1930's will differ from the real figures. The 5-year age groups for ages under 30 for each country are given in Appendix VII, Table A-VII-1. The hypothetical "B" populations (total, male and female, by age groups) for the eleven Latin American countries combined are given in Tables VIII-2, VIII-3, and VIII-4. For individual countries, see Appendix VIII, Table A-VIII-1.

The Effect on Population Growth

One of every four persons in Latin America in the 1960's would not have existed had fertility declined from the 1930's in such a way that crude birth rates followed the European relationship between birth rate and life expectancy (equation VIII-1). If the comparison is applied solely to those ages affected by the fertility decline (ages under 30), nearly 36 persons of each 100 would not have existed. If only the youngest ages are considered (0 to 4), more than half of the population enumerated in the 1960's would not have existed (Tables VIII-2, VIII-3, and VIII-4; see individual countries in Appendix VIII, Table A-VIII-1). The total population growth rate today would have been only 13 per thousand instead of the actual 32 per thousand. Such different growth rates result in completely different population sizes after several years. The disparity is shown in Table VIII-5, where the actual and hypothetical "B" populations in the 1960's are projected into the future, on the hypothesis that all conditions remain as they were in the 1960's.

From an economic point of view, the hypothetical "B" population growth rates would have been more favorable than the actual rates. With lower growth rates, economic efforts to maintain or increase the per capita income could have been less than what was actually required. Or the expended efforts could have been applied, perhaps with greater success, to a more favorable economic situation. I will not focus on this aspect of population growth in this study, however, but rather on the changes in the age structure of populations and the question of whether these changes were favorable to the welfare of the population.

The Effect of the Age Structure Change

If fertility had declined in actual Latin American populations at the rate of the hypothetical "B" projection from the

Table VIII-1

HYPOTHETICAL CRUDE BIRTH RATES USED FOR PROJECTED LATIN AMERICAN POPULATIONS: 1930's TO 1960's[a]

(per thousand)

	Years						
Country	1930	1935	1940	1945	1950	1955	1960
Brazil	42.0	40.7	38.9	36.4	33.2	29.1	24.5
Chile	40.4	39.5	37.5	33.6	28.4	25.4	24.0
Costa Rica[b]	32.7	30.1	27.7	25.4	23.4	21.8	20.6
El Salvador[c]	46.6	41.1	36.4	32.5	29.3	26.5	24.3
Guatemala[d]	50.7	46.7	41.5	36.1	31.5	28.3	27.1
Honduras[c]	41.3	39.5	37.7	35.5	32.7	29.3	25.4
Mexico	41.8	39.7	36.9	33.4	29.6	26.0	23.2
Nicaragua[b]	44.7	42.7	39.6	36.9	33.8	30.4	26.7
Panama	39.7	36.5	33.6	30.9	27.9	24.8	21.6
Paraguay[e]	40.0	37.7	35.2	32.5	29.8	27.1	24.4
Venezuela[c]	42.7	41.8	35.8	30.0	25.5	22.4	20.9
Average[f]	42.1	39.6	36.4	33.0	29.6	26.5	23.9

[a]The hypothetical crude birth rates are those that Latin American countries would have had if they had had the same birth rates as European countries at the same mortality level.

[b]1933, 1938, ... 1963

[c]1931, 1936, ... 1961

[d]1934, 1939, ... 1964

[e]1932, 1937, ... 1962

[f]The average is non-weighted.

Table VIII-2

ACTUAL AND HYPOTHETICAL "B" POPULATIONS, BOTH SEXES, IN ELEVEN LATIN AMERICAN COUNTRIES COMBINED: 1960's

(thousands)

	Populations		Differences		
	Actual	Hypothetical "B"[a]	Absolute (1)-(2)	Relative (3)÷(1)	Percent Distribution Column (3)
Age	(1)	(2)	(3)	(4)	(5)
Total	136,937.9	101,463.9	35,474.0	25.9	100.0
0- 4	24,557.0	10,965.9	13,591.1	55.3	38.3
5- 9	20,279.9	10,735.0	9,544.9	47.1	26.9
10-14	16,600.8	10,587.3	6,013.5	36.2	17.0
15-19	13,885.1	10,271.4	3,613.7	26.0	10.2
20-24	11,570.5	9,715.5	1,855.0	16.0	5.2
25-29	9,832.7	8,976.9	855.8	8.7	2.4
30-49	26,443.3[b]	26,443.3[b]			
50-64	9,698.9	9,698.9			
65+	4,069.7	4,069.7			
0-30	96,726.0	61,252.0	35,474.0	36.7	100.0

[a]The hypothetical "B" population is the population projected from the 1930's to the 1960's by using the hypothetical crude birth rates of Table VIII-1.

[b]The population over age 30 is the same in both populations and equal to that of Chapter V, Table V-4, Column (1).

Table VIII-3

ACTUAL AND HYPOTHETICAL "B" MALE POPULATIONS IN ELEVEN LATIN AMERICAN COUNTRIES COMBINED: 1960's

(thousands)

	Populations		Differences		
	Actual	Hypothetical "B"	Absolute (1)-(2)	Relative (3)÷(1)	Percent Distribution Column (3)
Age	(1)	(2)	(3)	(4)	(5)
Total	68,310.1	50,435.1	17,875.0	26.2	100.0
0- 4	12,509.7	5,584.1	6,925.6	55.4	38.7
5- 9	10,247.4	5,421.3	4,826.1	47.1	27.0
10-14	8,289.1	5,283.0	3,006.1	36.3	16.8
15-19	6,866.2	5,076.1	1,790.1	26.1	10.0
20-24	5,659.1	4,750.3	908.8	16.1	5.1
25-29	4,796.3	4,378.0	418.3	8.7	2.3
30-49	13,097.0[a]	13,097.0[a]			
50-64	4,884.9	4,884.9			
65+	1,960.4	1,960.4			
0-30	48,367.8	30,492.8	17,875.0	37.0	100.0

[a]The population over age 30 is the same in both populations and equal to that of Chapter V, Appendix V, Table A-V-2, Column (1).

Table VIII-4

ACTUAL AND HYPOTHETICAL "B" FEMALE POPULATIONS IN ELEVEN LATIN AMERICAN COUNTRIES COMBINED: 1960's

(thousands)

	Populations		Differences		
	Actual	Hypothetical "B"	Absolute (1)-(2)	Relative (3)÷(1)	Percent Distribution Column (3)
Age	(1)	(2)	(3)	(4)	(5)
Total	68,627.8	51,029.0	17,598.8	25.6	100.0
0- 4	12,047.3	5,381.7	6,665.6	55.3	37.9
5- 9	10,032.5	5,313.7	4,718.8	47.0	26.8
10-14	8,311.7	5,304.5	3,007.2	36.2	17.1
15-19	7,018.9	5,195.3	1,823.6	26.0	10.4
20-24	5,911.4	4,965.2	946.2	16.0	5.4
25-29	5,036.4	4,599.0	437.4	8.7	2.5
30-49	13,346.3[a]	13,346.3[a]			
50-64	4,814.0	4,814.0			
65+	2,109.3	2,109.3			
0-30	48,358.2	30,759.4	17,598.8	36.4	100.0

[a]The population over age 30 is the same in both populations and equal to that of Chapter V, Appendix V, Table A-V-2, Column (1).

Table VIII-5

ACTUAL AND HYPOTHETICAL "B" POPULATIONS, BOTH SEXES, IN ELEVEN LATIN AMERICAN COUNTRIES COMBINED: 1930-2020[a]

(thousands)

	Populations	
Year	Actual[b]	Hypothetical "B"[c]
1930	71,048.8	71,048.8
1950	102,986.5	86,853.7
1960	136,937.9	101,463.6
1990	355,145.3	150,258.9
2020	922,665.7	222,520.6

[a]The countries included are Brazil, Chile, Costa Rica, El Salvador, Guatemala, Honduras, Mexico, Nicaragua, Panama, Paraguay and Venezuela.

[b]Actual populations for 1930, 1950, and 1960. The populations for 1990 and 2020 were projected on the assumption that the population will grow at an annual geometric rate of 31.8 per thousand.

[c]From 1930 to 1960, populations are projected with the same mortality and birth rates as those of Europe at the same mortality level. After 1960, they are projected at a constant growth rate of 13.0 per thousand, which was the growth rate in 1955-1960.

1930's to the 1960's, the age structure of the population would have changed tremendously: only the population under age 30 would have decreased. As a consequence, the mean age of the population would have increased and the proportion of the population of non-active ages would have fallen.

For the eleven countries combined, the increase of the mean age of the population would have been 5.4 years. Instead of the 22.2 years mean age of the actual population, the mean age would have been 27.4 years. All the countries except Chile would have increased their mean ages by more than four years, with the range of change varying from 3.1 to 8.5 years for Chile and Costa Rica, respectively (see Table VIII-6).

Although the population would have been reduced only in the ages under 30, the proportional age group distribution would

Table VIII-6

MEAN AGE OF ACTUAL AND HYPOTHETICAL "B" POPULATIONS OF ELEVEN LATIN AMERICAN COUNTRIES: 1960's

	Total			Male			Female		
Country	Actual	Hypothetical "B"	Difference	Actual	Hypothetical "B"	Difference	Actual	Hypothetical "B"	Difference
Brazil	22.52	26.68	4.16	22.47	26.68	4.21	22.56	26.68	4.12
Chile	24.79	27.87	3.08	24.39	27.48	3.09	25.18	28.24	3.06
Costa Rica	21.33	29.83	8.50	21.23	29.79	8.56	21.43	29.88	8.45
El Salvador	21.92	27.36	5.44	21.59	27.06	5.47	22.24	27.65	5.40
Guatemala	21.60	26.50	4.90	21.55	26.49	4.94	21.65	26.51	4.86
Honduras	21.06	26.76	5.70	20.82	26.53	5.71	21.30	26.98	5.68
Mexico	22.11	27.97	5.86	21.80	27.70	5.90	21.41	28.24	6.83
Nicaragua	21.17	26.12	4.95	20.72	25.67	4.98	21.61	26.54	4.93
Panama	23.35	28.39	5.04	23.50	28.55	5.05	23.19	28.22	5.03
Paraguay	22.79	27.75	4.96	22.32	27.27	4.95	23.25	28.22	4.97
Venezuela	21.67	28.21	6.54	21.54	28.00	6.46	21.81	28.43	6.62
Average[a]	22.21	27.59	5.38	21.99	27.38	5.39	22.33	27.78	5.45

[a]The average is non-weighted.

have changed in all ages. The percentage changes in the populations for the eleven countries combined would have been as follows:

	Populations		
Age Group	Actual	Hypothetical "B"	Differences
Total	100.0	100.0	0.0
0-14	44.8	31.8	13.0
15-49	45.1	54.6	-9.5
50-64	7.1	9.6	-2.5
65+	3.0	4.0	-1.0

(For each 5-year age group and sex, see Table VIII-7. Details by country can be seen in Appendix VIII, Table A-VIII-2.)

Some Consequences of the Hypothetical Age Structure Changes

As we saw in Chapter VI, the principal consequences of age structure change are those related to the labor force and the cost of education. We shall deal with these consequences in the following pages.

Consequences for the Labor Force. The hypothetical "B" populations in the 1960's would have been smaller than the actual populations only in ages under 30. Thus, although the numbers in economically active ages would have been practically unchanged, the number of young dependent on them would have declined. For instance, the hypothetical "B" population of ages 15-64 for the eleven Latin American countries combined would have been 65.1 million instead of the actual 71.4 million--a reduction of only 8.9 percent. On the other hand, the population aged 0-14 plus those 65 and over would have been reduced from 65.5 to 36.4 million--that is, by 44.5 percent.[6]

[6] The change in the labor force would have been almost the same as in ages 15-64. Although some participation rates start at very young ages, the activity rates under age 15 are low. In order to get an idea of the change in the labor force that would have occurred, the labor forces in the actual and hypothetical populations were calculated by using the same age-specific labor

Table VIII-7

PROPORTIONAL AGE DISTRIBUTION IN ACTUAL AND HYPOTHETICAL "B" POPULATIONS OF ELEVEN LATIN AMERICAN COUNTRIES COMBINED: 1960's

(percentages)

	Totals		Male		Female	
Age Group	Actual	Hypothetical "B"	Actual	Hypothetical "B"	Actual	Hypothetical "B"
Total	100.000	100.000	100.000	100.000	100.000	100.000
0- 4	17.933	10.807	18.313	11.072	17.555	10.546
5- 9	14.810	10.580	15.001	10.749	14.619	10.413
10-14	12.123	10.435	12.135	10.475	12.111	10.395
15-19	10.140	10.123	10.052	10.065	10.227	10.181
20-24	8.449	9.575	8.284	9.419	8.614	9.730
25-29	7.180	8.847	7.021	8.680	7.339	9.013
30-34	6.123	8.264	6.018	8.151	6.227	8.375
35-39	5.207	7.027	5.147	6.971	5.266	7.082
40-44	4.356	5.879	4.359	5.904	4.352	5.854
45-49	3.625	4.892	3.648	4.940	3.602	4.844
50-54	2.926	3.949	2.955	4.002	2.898	3.897
55-59	2.345	3.165	2.370	3.206	2.320	3.120
60-64	1.811	2.445	1.825	2.474	1.797	2.416
65-69	1.327	1.791	1.328	1.798	1.326	1.784
70-74	.864	1.166	.845	1.145	.882	1.186
75-79	.434	.585	.402	.544	.465	.626
80-84	.207	.279	.182	.246	.232	.312
85+	.141	.190	.114	.154	.168	.226
0-14	44.865	31.822	45.449	32.296	44.285	31.355
15-49	45.080	54.607	44.530	54.132	45.627	55.078
50-64	7.083	9.559	7.151	9.686	7.015	9.434
65+	2.972	4.011	2.870	3.887	3.074	4.134

Source: Tables VIII-2, VIII-3, and VIII-4.

This fact deserves emphasis. Even in the hypothetical "B" case, where fertility would have declined at an extremely rapid pace (almost as quickly as mortality), the population in the active ages, even after three decades of decline, would have been only very slightly reduced. The countries would have had manpower for economic development, without overloading it with an increased number of dependents. Thus, on the reasonable assumption that national income is produced by the economically active population, the national income would have remained the same, because this population would not have changed. Therefore, the real per capita income in the 1960's would have been 35 percent greater than it was. If consumer behavior had remained constant, such an increase of per capita income--or a great proportion of it--could have been saved and probably invested. If such investments had been adequate, there is no doubt that these countries would have been much better off than they actually were in the 1960's.[7] If fertility had declined, the populations would have escaped the tremendous burden of the large non-economically active population which existed in the 1960's.

In order to examine the situation more closely, the dependency ratios of the actual and hypothetical "B" populations have been calculated in Table VIII-8. In the hypothetical population, on the average, each person between ages 15-64 would have had .3 less dependents. The figure is .5 dependents for persons aged 20-64. The number of dependents per worker would have declined about .7 (see Table VIII-9), and the total activity rates of the populations (in hundreds) would have increased eight points (see Table VIII-10). All these changes related to labor force would have occurred if fertility had declined and all other variables had remained the same.

---

force participation rates. I chose the 1960 Mexican census participation rates (from United Nations, Demographic Yearbook 1964 [New York, 1965], p. 203) as standard because these rates start at the very young age of 8 and give maximum differences. The labor force of the eleven Latin American countries combined was 44.1 million in the actual population and 40.0 million in the hypothetical population, a reduction of 9.2 percent.

[7]It can be argued that production would have declined because of a reduction in the demand for goods, which would have followed upon the decline in the proportion of the population under age 30, most of whom are consumers. We cannot discuss this issue here, except to point out that an increase of the market would have been possible. Although the population would have been smaller, a greater number of people would have participated in the market because of increased income.

Table VIII-8

DEPENDENCY RATIOS OF ACTUAL AND HYPOTHETICAL "B" POPULATIONS, BOTH SEXES, IN ELEVEN LATIN AMERICAN COUNTRIES: 1960's

		Dependency Ratios			
		$\frac{N_{0-14}+N_{65+}}{N_{15-64}}$		$\frac{N_{0-19}+N_{65+}}{N_{20-64}}$	
Country	Year	Actual	Hypothetical "B"	Actual	Hypothetical "B"
Brazil	1960	.89	.57	1.34	.88
Chile	1960	.80	.56	1.18	.85
Costa Rica	1963	1.06	.48	1.60	.71
El Salvador	1961	.99	.55	1.48	.83
Guatemala	1964	.98	.56	1.47	.87
Honduras	1961	1.02	.57	1.54	.86
Mexico	1960	.96	.55	1.45	.82
Nicaragua	1963	1.04	.60	1.58	.93
Panama	1960	.88	.54	1.32	.81
Paraguay	1962	.96	.58	1.46	.88
Venezuela	1961	.97	.48	1.44	.73
Average[a]		.89	.56	1.35	.85

[a]The average is non-weighted.

Table VIII-9

RATIO OF NON-ACTIVE TO ACTIVE POPULATION IN ACTUAL AND HYPOTHETICAL "B" POPULATIONS IN SELECTED LATIN AMERICAN COUNTRIES: 1960's

	Totals		Male		Female	
Country	Actual	Hypothetical "B"[a]	Actual	Hypothetical "B"	Actual	Hypothetical "B"
Chile	2.10	1.68	.96	.69	6.08	5.17
Costa Rica	2.41	1.47	1.04	.46	9.43	6.94
El Salvador	2.20	1.53	.93	.51	8.01	6.23
Honduras	2.31	1.64	.89	.50	11.94	9.60
Mexico	2.15	1.48	.91	.50	7.85	5.95
Nicaragua	2.21	1.56	.98	.57	7.06	5.43
Panama	2.00	1.45	.94	.58	5.90	4.71
Venezuela	2.23	1.42	1.02	.51	7.50	5.50
Average[b]	2.20	1.53	.96	.54	7.97	6.19

[a] Actual age-specific activity rates were applied to the hypothetical population (Appendix VIII, Table A-VIII-1). Age-specific activity rates are from United Nations, Demographic Yearbook 1964 (New York, 1965), Table 8.

[b] The average is non-weighted.

Table VIII-10

TOTAL ACTIVITY RATES OF ACTUAL AND HYPOTHETICAL "B" POPULATIONS IN SELECTED LATIN AMERICAN POPULATIONS: 1960's[a]

Country	Totals		Male		Female	
	Actual	Hypothetical "B"	Actual	Hypothetical "B"	Actual	Hypothetical "B"
Chile	32.3	37.3	51.1	59.3	14.1	16.2
Costa Rica	29.4	40.4	49.0	68.3	9.6	12.6
El Salvador	31.2	39.5	51.9	66.2	11.1	13.8
Honduras	30.2	37.8	52.8	66.7	7.7	9.4
Mexico	31.8	40.3	52.3	66.6	11.3	14.4
Nicaragua	31.2	39.1	50.4	63.6	12.4	15.6
Panama	33.3	40.9	51.5	63.3	14.5	17.5
Venezuela	30.9	41.3	49.5	66.3	11.8	15.4
Average[b]	31.3	39.6	51.1	65.0	11.6	14.4

[a]Total activity rates are defined as the ratio of the active population to the total population. The rates for the hypothetical population were found by applying the actual age-specific activity rates to the hypothetical populations of Appendix VIII, Table A-VIII-1. Actual age-specific activity rates are from United Nations, Demographic Yearbook 1964 (New York, 1965), Table 8.

[b]The average is non-weighted.

Consequences for the Cost of Education. As for costs of education, a very favorable state for educational improvement would have been reached under hypothetical "B" population conditions in the 1960's. The population under age 15 per worker was 1.394 in the actual population and only .807 in the hypothetical "B" population. If educational cost per student and assistance rate remained constant, the cost of education per worker would have been reduced by 42 percent. Or, better still, the expenditures for education per student could have been raised by 42 percent without extra cost to the nation.

Conclusions

If from the 1930's to the 1960's fertility in Latin American countries had declined as it did in Europe when an equal mortality level existed, the economic situation in those countries in the 1960's would have been markedly better than it was. The situation would probably have been even much better than the hypothetical "B" case presented here. The number of children per woman would have been smaller: women would have stopped having babies at early ages, or started at older ages, or had them at more widely spaced intervals. In the first two cases women would have been able to participate in the labor force, and contribute to economic development. Thus, a labor force greater than the one that actually existed would have been likely.

The reader may question whether such a decline of fertility was possible. The answer to this question, given in the next chapter, must take into account a variable which up to now has been left out: time.

APPENDIX VIII

Table A-VIII-1

ACTUAL AND HYPOTHETICAL "B" POPULATIONS IN ELEVEN LATIN AMERICAN COUNTRIES: 1960's

(thousands)

BRAZIL

	Populations		Differences		Percent Distribution of the Difference
	Actual	Hypothetical "B"	Absolute (1)-(2)	Relative (3)÷(1)	(3) ÷ 8,268.3
Age	(1)	(2)	(3)	(4)	(5)
			Male		
Total	35,808.2	27,539.9	8,268.3	23.1	100.0
0- 4	6,392.1	3,115.8	3,276.3	51.3	39.6
5- 9	5,317.3	3,043.4	2,273.9	42.8	27.5
10-14	4,306.7	2,946.5	1,360.2	31.6	16.5
15-19	3,589.4	2,797.5	791.9	22.1	9.6
20-24	2,988.0	2,593.5	394.5	13.2	4.8
25-29	2,551.6	2,380.1	171.5	6.7	2.1
30-49	7,065.2	7,065.2			
50-64	2,606.8	2,606.8			
65+	991.1	991.1			
0-30	25,145.1	16,876.8	8,268.3	32.9	100.0
			Female		
					(3) ÷ 8,196.5
Total	35,971.4	27,774.9	8,196.5	22.8	100.0
0- 4	6,163.4	3,004.4	3,159.0	51.3	38.5
5- 9	5,242.2	3,000.5	2,241.7	42.8	27.3
10-14	4,366.3	2,987.3	1,379.0	31.6	16.8
15-19	3,716.3	2,896.4	819.9	22.1	10.0
20-24	3,150.4	2,734.5	415.9	13.2	5.1
25-29	2,693.9	2,512.9	181.0	6.7	2.2
30-49	7,127.6	7,127.6			
50-64	2,478.0	2,478.0			
65+	1,033.3	1,033.3			
0-30	25,332.5	17,136.0	8,196.5	32.4	100.0

APPENDIX VIII

Table A-VIII-1 (continued)

CHILE

Age	Populations: Actual (1)	Populations: Hypothetical "B" (2)	Differences: Absolute (1)-(2) (3)	Differences: Relative (3)÷(1) (4)	Percent Distribution of the Difference (3) ÷ 522.9 (5)
			Male		
Total	3,634.5	3,111.6	522.9	14.4	100.0
0- 4	582.0	334.6	247.4	42.5	47.3
5- 9	492.4	327.4	165.0	33.5	31.6
10-14	417.3	324.9	92.4	22.1	17.7
15-19	357.0	319.9	37.1	10.4	7.1
20-24	301.2	302.2	-1.0	-.3	-.2
25-29	261.8	279.8	-18.0	-6.9	-3.4
30-49	765.1	765.1			
50-64	321.3	321.3			
65+	136.4	136.4			
0-30	2,411.7	1,888.8	522.9	21.7	100.0
			Female		
					(3) ÷ 520.2
Total	3,776.6	3,256.4	520.2	13.8	100.0
0- 4	575.8	331.1	244.7	42.5	47.0
5- 9	489.0	325.1	163.9	33.5	31.5
10-14	423.2	329.5	93.7	22.1	18.0
15-19	368.2	330.0	38.2	10.4	7.3
20-24	318.0	319.1	-1.1	-.3	-.2
25-29	279.7	298.9	-19.2	-6.9	-3.7
30-49	815.7	815.7			
50-64	340.9	340.9			
65+	166.1	166.1			
0-30	2,453.9	1,933.7	520.2	21.2	100.0

APPENDIX VIII

Table A-VIII-1 (continued)

COSTA RICA

	Populations		Differences		Percent Distribution of the Difference
	Actual	Hypothetical "B"	Absolute (1)-(2)	Relative (3)÷(1)	(3) ÷ 287.5
Age	(1)	(2)	(3)	(4)	(5)
			Male		
Total	679.2	391.7	287.5	42.3	100.0
0- 4	137.1	37.3	99.8	72.8	34.7
5- 9	110.5	36.1	74.4	67.3	25.9
10-14	84.7	35.1	49.6	58.6	17.3
15-19	67.7	34.5	33.2	49.0	11.5
20-24	53.0	33.6	19.4	36.6	6.7
25-29	43.9	32.8	11.1	25.3	3.9
30-49	117.0	117.0			
50-64	44.5	44.5			
65+	20.8	20.8			
0-30	496.9	209.4	287.5	57.9	100.0
			Female		
					(3) ÷ 283.3
Total	676.5	393.2	283.3	41.9	100.0
0- 4	133.0	36.2	96.8	72.8	34.2
5- 9	107.1	35.0	72.1	67.3	25.5
10-14	84.4	35.0	49.4	58.5	17.4
15-19	68.3	34.8	33.5	49.0	11.8
20-24	54.6	34.6	20.0	36.6	7.1
25-29	45.2	33.7	11.5	25.4	4.1
30-49	119.0	119.0			
50-64	44.4	44.4			
65+	20.5	20.5			
0-30	492.6	209.3	283.3	57.5	100.0

APPENDIX VIII

Table A-VIII-1 (continued)

EL SALVADOR

	Populations		Differences		Percent Distribution of the Difference
	Actual	Hypothetical "B"	Absolute (1)-(2)	Relative (3)÷(1)	(3) ÷ 362.8
Age	(1)	(2)	(3)	(4)	(5)
			Male		
Total	1,271.7	908.9	362.8	28.5	100.0
0- 4	247.6	100.5	147.1	59.4	40.5
5- 9	200.8	96.3	104.5	52.0	28.8
10-14	156.8	94.4	62.4	39.8	17.2
15-19	126.9	92.0	34.9	27.5	9.6
20-24	102.0	88.3	13.7	13.4	3.8
25-29	85.0	84.8	.2	.2	.1
30-49	229.2	229.2			
50-64	86.4	86.4			
65+	37.0	37.0			
0-30	919.1	556.3	362.8	39.5	100.0
			Female		
					(3) ÷ 360.1
Total	1,307.7	947.6	360.1	27.5	100.0
0- 4	242.0	98.3	143.7	59.4	39.9
5- 9	198.3	95.1	103.2	52.0	28.7
10-14	157.2	94.6	62.6	39.8	17.4
15-19	130.1	94.3	35.8	27.5	9.9
20-24	108.5	93.9	14.6	13.5	4.1
25-29	92.3	92.1	.2	.2	.1
30-49	247.9	247.9			
50-64	90.1	90.1			
65+	41.3	41.3			
0-30	928.4	568.3	360.1	38.8	100.0

APPENDIX VIII

Table A-VIII-1 (continued)

GUATEMALA

Age	Populations: Actual (1)	Populations: Hypothetical "B" (2)	Differences: Absolute (1)-(2) (3)	Differences: Relative (3)÷(1) (4)	Percent Distribution of the Difference (3) ÷ 562.4 (5)
			Male		
Total	2,135.7	1,573.3	562.4	26.3	100.0
0- 4	410.5	180.9	229.6	55.9	40.8
5- 9	333.9	168.1	165.8	49.7	29.5
10-14	262.0	166.0	96.0	36.6	17.1
15-19	214.5	163.2	51.3	23.9	9.1
20-24	174.4	155.5	18.9	10.8	3.4
25-29	146.7	145.9	.8	.5	.1
30-49	395.6	395.6			
50-64	140.9	140.9			
65+	57.2	57.2			
0-30	1,542.0	979.6	562.4	36.5	100.0
			Female		
					(3) ÷ 558.6
Total	2,145.1	1,586.5	558.6	26.0	100.0
0- 4	403.7	177.9	225.8	55.9	40.4
5- 9	330.8	166.6	164.2	49.6	29.4
10-14	262.4	166.2	96.2	36.7	17.2
15-19	217.0	165.1	51.9	23.9	3.5
20-24	181.2	161.6	19.6	10.8	3.5
25-29	153.1	152.2	.9	.6	.2
30-49	400.3	400.3			
50-64	139.9	139.9			
65+	56.7	56.7			
0-30	1,548.2	989.6	558.6	36.1	100.0

APPENDIX VIII

Table A-VIII-1 (continued)

HONDURAS

	Populations		Differences		Percent Distribution of
	Actual	Hypothetical "B"	Absolute (1)-(2)	Relative (3)÷(1)	the Difference (3) ÷ 306.7
Age	(1)	(2)	(3)	(4)	(5)
			Male		
Total	937.4	630.7	306.7	32.7	100.0
0- 4	186.2	72.6	113.6	61.0	37.0
5- 9	151.3	69.9	81.4	53.8	26.5
10-14	118.5	67.5	51.0	43.0	16.6
15-19	95.9	63.6	32.3	33.7	10.5
20-24	77.0	58.5	18.5	24.0	6.0
25-29	63.7	53.8	9.9	15.5	3.2
30-49	164.7	164.7			
50-64	58.2	58.2			
65+	21.9	21.9			
0-30	692.6	385.9	306.7	44.3	100.0
			Female		
					(3) ÷ 302.4
Total	944.0	641.6	302.4	32.0	100.0
0- 4	179.4	69.9	109.5	61.0	36.2
5- 9	148.6	68.7	79.9	53.8	26.4
10-14	117.7	67.0	50.7	43.1	16.8
15-19	97.0	64.3	32.7	33.7	10.8
20-24	80.0	60.8	19.2	24.0	6.3
25-29	67.0	56.6	10.4	15.5	3.4
30-49	171.0	171.0			
50-64	58.9	58.9			
65+	24.4	24.4			
0-30	689.7	387.3	302.4	33.5	100.0

APPENDIX VIII

Table A-VIII-1 (continued)

MEXICO

	Populations		Differences		Percent Distribution of the Difference
	Actual	Hypothetical "B"	Absolute (1)-(2)	Relative (3)÷(1)	(3) ÷ 5,696.0
Age	(1)	(2)	(3)	(4)	(5)
			Male		
Total	17,812.7	12,116.7	5,696.0	32.0	100.0
0- 4	3,407.5	1,316.4	2,091.1	61.4	36.7
5- 9	2,716.0	1,265.5	1,450.5	53.4	25.5
10-14	2,209.3	1,235.8	973.5	44.1	17.1
15-19	1,812.5	1,193.3	619.2	34.2	10.8
20-24	1,468.3	1,113.1	355.2	24.2	6.2
25-29	1,223.7	1,017.2	206.5	16.9	3.6
30-49	3,211.2	3,211.2			
50-64	1,222.8	1,222.8			
65+	541.4	541.4			
0-30	12,837.1	7,141.3	5,696.0	44.4	100.0
			Female		
					(3) ÷ 5,559.9
Total	17,880.4	12,320.5	5,559.9	31.1	100.0
0- 4	3,238.7	1,251.2	1,987.5	61.4	35.7
5- 9	2,618.4	1,220.1	1,398.3	53.4	25.1
10-14	2,181.4	1,220.2	961.2	44.1	17.3
15-19	1,829.2	1,204.3	624.9	34.2	11.2
20-24	1,529.2	1,159.2	370.0	24.2	6.7
25-29	1,291.3	1,073.3	218.0	16.9	3.9
30-49	3,354.5	3,354.5			
50-64	1,259.4	1,259.4			
65+	578.3	578.3			
0-30	12,688.2	7,128.3	5,559.9	43.8	100.0

Table A-VIII-1 (continued)

NICARAGUA

	Populations		Differences		Percent Distribution of the Difference
	Actual	Hypothetical "B"	Absolute (1)-(2)	Relative (3)÷(1)	(3) ÷ 207.6
Age	(1)	(2)	(3)	(4)	(5)
			Male		
Total	756.4	548.8	207.6	27.4	100.0
0- 4	152.8	66.1	86.7	56.7	41.8
5- 9	123.5	63.1	60.4	48.9	29.1
10-14	96.1	61.0	35.1	36.5	16.9
15-19	77.3	58.3	19.0	24.6	9.2
20-24	61.7	54.8	6.9	11.2	3.3
25-29	50.7	51.3	-.6	-1.2	-.3
30-49	129.2	129.2			
50-64	45.1	45.1			
65+	20.0	20.0			
0-30	562.1	354.6	207.6	36.9	100.0
			Female		
					(3) ÷ 204.0
Total	775.8	571.8	204.0	26.3	100.0
0- 4	146.4	63.3	83.1	56.8	40.7
5- 9	120.9	61.8	59.1	48.9	29.0
10-14	96.9	61.5	35.4	36.5	17.3
15-19	79.9	60.3	19.6	24.5	9.6
20-24	65.7	58.3	7.4	11.3	3.6
25-29	54.9	55.6	-.7	-1.3	-.3
30-49	138.5	138.5			
50-64	48.3	48.3			
65+	24.3	24.3			
0-30	564.7	360.8	204.0	36.1	100.0

APPENDIX VIII

Table A-VIII-1 (continued)

PANAMA

	Populations		Differences		Percent Distribution of the Difference
	Actual	Hypothetical "B"	Absolute (1)-(2)	Relative (3)÷(1)	(3) ÷ 134.7
Age	(1)	(2)	(3)	(4)	(5)
			Male		
Total	515.1	380.4	134.7	26.2	100.0
0- 4	86.1	38.0	48.1	55.9	35.7
5- 9	73.3	37.8	35.5	48.4	26.4
10-14	61.1	37.4	23.7	38.9	17.6
15-19	51.7	36.4	15.3	29.6	11.4
20-24	43.1	34.9	8.2	19.0	6.1
25-29	37.1	33.3	3.8	10.2	2.8
30-49	104.5	104.5			
50-64	39.6	39.6			
65+	18.6	18.6			
0-30	352.4	217.8	134.6	38.2	100.0
			Female		
					(3) ÷ 131.5
Total	496.5	365.0	131.5	28.3	100.0
0- 4	83.7	36.9	48.8	55.9	37.1
5- 9	71.6	36.9	34.7	48.5	26.3
10-14	59.9	36.7	23.2	38.7	17.6
15-19	50.8	35.8	15.0	29.5	11.4
20-24	42.4	34.3	8.1	19.1	6.2
25-29	36.1	32.4	11.8	32.7	9.0
30-49	97.7	97.7			
50-64	36.2	36.2			
65+	18.1	18.1			
0-30	344.5	213.0	131.5	38.3	100.0

APPENDIX VIII

Table A-VIII-1 (continued)

PARAGUAY

	Populations		Differences		Percent Distribution of
	Actual	Hypothetical "B"	Absolute (1)-(2)	Relative (3)÷(1)	the Difference (3) ÷ 232.4
Age	(1)	(2)	(3)	(4)	(5)
			Male		
Total	893.3	660.9	232.4	26.0	100.0
0- 4	161.7	73.7	88.0	54.4	37.9
5- 9	137.1	71.2	65.9	48.1	28.3
10-14	113.3	70.0	43.3	38.2	18.6
15-19	93.6	67.8	25.8	27.6	11.1
20-24	73.7	64.2	9.5	12.9	4.1
25-29	60.5	60.6	-.1	-.2	-.1
30-49	156.1	156.1			
50-64	64.5	64.5			
65+	32.8	32.8			
0-30	639.9	407.5	232.4	36.3	100.0
			Female		
					(3) ÷ 227.2
Total	910.5	683.3	227.2	25.0	100.0
0- 4	157.4	71.7	85.7	54.4	37.7
5- 9	133.5	69.3	64.2	48.1	28.3
10-14	110.5	68.2	42.3	38.3	18.6
15-19	92.6	67.1	25.5	27.5	11.2
20-24	75.6	65.9	9.7	12.8	4.3
25-29	63.6	63.7	-.1	-.2	.0
30-49	172.0	172.0			
50-64	67.7	67.7			
65+	37.6	37.6			
0-30	633.2	405.9	227.3	35.9	100.0

APPENDIX VIII

Table A-VIII-1 (continued)

VENEZUELA

	Populations		Differences		Percent Distribution of the Difference
	Actual	Hypothetical "B"	Absolute (1)-(2)	Relative (3)÷(1)	(3) ÷ 1,294.0
Age	(1)	(2)	(3)	(4)	(5)
			Male		
Total	3,865.9	2,571.9	1,294.0	33.5	100.0
0- 4	746.1	248.2	497.9	66.7	38.5
5- 9	591.3	242.5	348.8	59.0	27.0
10-14	463.3	244.4	218.9	47.2	16.9
15-19	379.7	249.6	130.1	32.3	10.1
20-24	316.7	251.7	65.0	20.5	5.0
25-29	271.6	238.4	33.2	12.2	25.7
30-49	759.2	759.2			
50-64	254.8	254.8			
65+	83.2	83.2			
0-30	2,768.7	1,474.8	1,293.9	46.7	100.0
			Female		
					(3) ÷ 1,255.1
Total	3,743.3	2,488.2	1,255.1	33.5	100.0
0- 4	723.8	240.8	483.0	66.7	38.5
5- 9	572.1	234.6	337.5	59.0	26.9
10-14	451.8	238.3	213.5	47.3	17.0
15-19	369.5	242.9	126.6	34.3	10.1
20-24	305.8	243.0	62.8	20.5	5.0
25-29	259.3	227.6	31.7	12.2	2.5
30-49	702.1	702.1			
50-64	250.2	250.2			
65+	108.7	108.7			
0-30	2,682.3	1,426.6	1,255.7	46.8	100.0

APPENDIX VIII

Table A-VIII-2

PROPORTIONAL AGE GROUP DISTRIBUTION OF THE ACTUAL AND HYPOTHETICAL "B" POPULATIONS IN ELEVEN LATIN AMERICAN COUNTRIES: 1960's

(percentages)

	Totals		Male		Female	
Age	Actual	Hypothetical "B"	Actual	Hypothetical "B"	Actual	Hypothetical "B"
			BRAZIL: 1960			
Total	100.000	100.000	100.000	100.000	100.000	100.000
0-14	44.286	32.718	44.727	33.064	43.846	32.375
15-49	45.810	54.430	45.225	53.872	46.393	54.983
50-64	7.084	9.192	7.280	9.465	6.889	8.922
65+	2.820	3.660	2.768	3.599	2.873	3.720
			CHILE: 1960			
Total	100.000	100.000	100.000	100.000	100.000	100.000
0-14	40.206	30.976	41.043	31.716	39.401	30.269
15-49	46.777	53.874	46.364	53.574	47.175	54.161
50-64	8.935	10.399	8.840	10.326	9.027	10.469
65+	4.082	4.750	3.753	4.384	4.398	5.101
			COSTA RICA: 1963			
Total	100.000	100.000	100.000	100.000	100.000	100.000
0-14	48.447	27.346	48.925	27.700	47.967	26.994
15-49	41.949	56.063	41.461	55.625	42.439	56.499
50-64	6.557	11.328	6.552	11.363	6.563	11.293
65+	3.046	5.263	3.062	5.311	3.030	5.214

APPENDIX VIII

Table A-VIII-2 (continued)

Age	Totals Actual	Totals Hypothetical "B"	Male Actual	Male Hypothetical "B"	Female Actual	Female Hypothetical "B"
			EL SALVADOR: 1961			
Total	100.000	100.000	100.000	100.000	100.000	100.000
0-14	46.627	31.205	47.590	32.047	45.691	30.397
15-49	43.495	55.071	42.707	54.377	44.261	55.737
50-64	6.843	9.507	6.794	9.506	6.890	9.508
65+	3.036	4.218	2.909	4.071	3.158	4.358
			GUATEMALA: 1964			
Total	100.000	100.000	100.000	100.000	100.000	100.000
0-14	46.797	32.459	47.123	32.733	46.473	32.189
15-49	43.982	55.049	43.602	54.676	44.362	55.419
50-64	6.560	8.887	6.597	8.956	6.522	8.818
65+	2.661	3.605	2.678	3.636	2.643	3.574
			HONDURAS: 1961			
Total	100.000	100.000	100.000	100.000	100.000	100.000
0-14	47.927	32.664	48.645	33.293	47.214	32.046
15-49	43.388	54.493	42.810	54.007	43.962	54.971
50-64	6.224	9.204	6.209	9.228	6.239	9.180
65+	2.461	3.639	2.336	3.472	2.585	3.803
			MEXICO: 1960			
Total	100.000	100.000	100.000	100.000	100.000	100.000
0-14	45.867	30.729	46.780	31.509	44.957	29.962
15-49	44.042	54.532	43.316	53.931	44.765	55.122
50-64	6.954	10.157	6.865	10.092	7.043	10.222
65+	3.137	4.582	3.039	4.468	3.234	4.694

APPENDIX VIII

Table A-VIII-2 (continued)

Age	Totals		Male		Female	
	Actual	Hypothet-ical "B"	Actual	Hypothet-ical "B"	Actual	Hypothet-ical "B"
			NICARAGUA: 1963			
Total	100.000	100.000	100.000	100.000	100.000	100.000
0-14	48.075	33.614	49.233	34.645	46.945	32.625
15-49	42.938	54.098	42.160	53.494	43.697	54.678
50-64	6.096	8.335	5.962	8.218	6.226	8.447
65+	2.891	3.953	2.644	3.644	3.132	4.250
			PANAMA: 1960			
Total	100.000	100.000	100.000	100.000	100.000	100.000
0-14	43.070	30.008	42.807	29.749	43.343	30.278
15-49	45.809	54.900	45.894	54.953	45.720	54.844
50-64	7.493	10.169	7.688	10.409	7.291	9.919
65+	3.628	4.923	3.611	4.889	3.646	4.959
			PARAGUAY: 1962			
Total	100.000	100.000	100.000	100.000	100.000	100.000
0-14	45.099	31.557	46.132	32.512	44.086	30.634
15-49	43.669	53.370	42.975	52.766	44.349	53.955
50-64	7.329	9.835	7.220	9.759	7.435	9.908
65+	3.903	5.237	3.672	4.963	4.130	5.503
			VENEZUELA: 1961			
Total	100.000	100.000	100.000	100.000	100.000	100.000
0-14	46.633	28.630	46.579	28.579	46.689	28.682
15-49	44.208	57.598	44.678	58.279	43.723	56.894
50-64	6.637	9.980	6.591	9.907	6.684	10.055
65+	2.522	3.792	2.152	3.235	2.904	4.369

Chapter IX

COULD LATIN AMERICA HAVE DUPLICATED THE EUROPEAN MORTALITY-FERTILITY MODEL?

The last two chapters show that Latin American fertility trends rose from the 1930's to the 1960's. The relationship between mortality and fertility in Latin America has been so different from that in European countries that one begins to believe that a duplication of the European fertility trend, in view of the rapid decline in mortality, was impossible. In this chapter we shall first determine the magnitude of the changes necessary for Latin American fertility to show the same relation to mortality that European fertility has shown. The possibility of such changes actually occurring, and by what means, will then be discussed. Finally, the crucial variable of time will be included in the analysis in order to explain what has actually happened.

Hypothetical Fertility in Latin American Countries: Europe as Model

Change of Birth Rates. Estimated crude birth rates in Latin America in the 1930's were approximately 42 per thousand; thirty years later, in order to reproduce the same mortality-fertility relationship shown by European countries, they should have been at a level lower than 24 per thousand (see Table IX-1). The hypothetical rates should have been only 56 percent of the levels exhibited in the 1930's. Birth rates in individual countries should have been from 37 to 54 percent lower than 1930's levels (Paraguay and Costa Rica, respectively).[1] In actuality, however, crude birth rates in the 1960's were, on the average, at an even higher level than in the 1930's--an incredible 45.5

---

[1]The crude birth rate of Paraguay in 1932 has probably been underestimated. The rate was calculated by rejuvenating the 1962 population; however, there had been considerable emigration from Paraguay during the preceding 30 years--principally during the decade just prior to the census. Therefore, the rejuvenated births of those enumerated are probably fewer than the births which actually occurred. The actual crude birth rate in 1932 may well have been higher, and therefore the 37 percent hypothetical decline given in the text is very likely an underestimate.

Table IX-1

COMPARISON OF ACTUAL CRUDE BIRTH RATES IN THE 1930's WITH HYPOTHETICAL CRUDE BIRTH RATES IN THE 1960's IN ELEVEN LATIN AMERICAN COUNTRIES

(rates per thousand)

	Rates		Differences	
	Actual 1930's[a]	Hypothetical 1960's[b]	Absolute (1)-(2)	Relative [(3)÷(1)] 100
Country	(1)	(2)	(3)	(4)
Brazil	44.1	24.5	19.5	44
Chile	40.2	24.0	16.2	40
Costa Rica	44.6	20.6	24.0	54
El Salvador	46.5	24.3	22.2	48
Guatemala	46.2	27.1	19.1	42
Honduras	42.0	25.4	16.6	40
Mexico	44.1	23.2	20.9	47
Nicaragua	42.9	26.7	16.2	38
Panama	37.4	21.6	15.8	42
Paraguay	38.8	24.4	14.4	37
Venezuela	39.9	20.9	16.0	40
Average	42.4	23.9	18.5	44

[a]From Table VII-2.

[b]Calculated by equation (IX-1) of the text.

per thousand. Instead of declining, fertility was further than ever from the hypothetical level (see Table IX-2).

Change of Age-Specific Fertility Rates. The hypothetical reduction of the birth rate implies a corresponding reduction in age-specific fertility rates, whose required theoretical decrease can be calculated by comparing the actual rates with those which would generate the hypothetical crude birth rates of the 1960's. The hypothetical age-specific fertility rates are not known, but it is reasonable to assume that their pattern[2] would have resembled the pattern of other countries with low fertility, such as European countries. Therefore, a pattern was derived by calculating the average age-specific fertility rates for several European countries--namely, Iceland, Ireland, Malta, the Netherlands, Portugal, and Yugoslavia--which were selected because they had crude birth rates similar to the hypothetical crude birth rates for Latin American countries in the 1960's (see Table IX-3). A proportional adjustment to this average set of rates was made for each Latin American country in order that the rates reproduce the country's hypothetical crude birth rate (see Table IX-4; for each country, see Appendix IX, Table A-IX-1).[3] The absolute difference between the actual and the hypothetical age-specific fertility rates gives the number of mothers per thousand females who would have avoided having children during a particular year if the mortality-fertility model had resembled the European model. The maximum is found in ages 20-24: on the average, 174 mothers per thousand females would not have had children. In individual countries, for the same age group, this number varies from 78 to 220 mothers per thousand females (Chile and Costa Rica, respectively; see Appendix IX, Table A-IX-1).

The relative difference of the age-specific fertility rates shows the number of mothers who would not have had children per thousand mothers. There is a maximum reduction at age 15 to

---

[2]By "pattern" is meant the relative relationship that the age-specific fertility rates have among themselves.

[3]The steps for adjusting the rates were: (a) the average set of age-specific fertility rates (Table IX-3) was applied to each Latin American country's hypothetical population in the 1960's--with the birth rate declining as in European countries at the same mortality level; (b) a crude birth rate was calculated from (a); (c) the hypothetical crude birth rate for each country (those of Table IX-1, Column 2) was divided by the rate calculated in (b); (d) each age-specific fertility rate of the "model" average set (Table IX-3) was multiplied by the ratio calculated in (c); (e) the resulting rate was assumed to pertain to each country.

Table IX-2

CRUDE BIRTH RATES FOR ACTUAL AND HYPOTHETICAL "B" POPULATIONS WITH CONSTANT AGE-SPECIFIC FERTILITY RATES IN ELEVEN LATIN AMERICAN COUNTRIES: 1960's

(per thousand)

		Birth Rates		Differences	
	Gross Reproduction Rate	Actual Population	Hypothetical "B" Population	Absolute (2)-(3)	Percent (4)÷(2)
Country	(1)	(2)	(3)	(4)	(5)
Brazil	2.99	44.0	24.5	19.5	44.3
Chile	2.48	37.1	24.0	13.1	35.3
Costa Rica	3.52	47.0	20.6	26.4	56.2
El Salvador	3.30	47.9	24.3	23.6	49.3
Guatemala	3.40	49.0	27.1	21.9	44.7
Honduras	3.49	49.7	25.4	24.3	48.9
Mexico	3.17	45.0	23.2	21.8	48.4
Nicaragua	3.45	50.6	26.7	23.9	47.2
Panama	2.68	40.3	21.6	18.7	46.4
Paraguay	3.15	44.0	24.4	19.6	44.5
Venezuela	3.31	46.1	20.9	25.2	54.7
Average	3.18	45.5	23.9	21.6	47.5

Table IX-3

AGE-SPECIFIC FERTILITY RATES FOR SELECTED EUROPEAN COUNTRIES: 1960

Country	Age Groups							Birth Rate
	15-19	20-24	25-29	30-34	35-39	40-44	45-49	
Iceland	.0389	.2407	.2085	.1592	.1051	.0423	.0032	28.0
Ireland[a]	.0042	.1082	.2169	.2095	.1522	.0577	.0042	21.4
Malta	.0093	.1981	.2008	.1504	.1050	.0418	.0053	26.1
Netherlands	.0072	.1218	.2076	.1532	.0883	.0338	.0028	20.8
Portugal	.0126	.1516	.1799	.1322	.0951	.0428	.0041	24.2
Yugoslavia[a]	.0225	.1791	.1548	.0909	.0491	.0253	.0056	23.5
Average	.0157	.1666	.1948	.1493	.0992	.0406	.0042	24.0

[a]Rates for 1961.

Source: United Nations, Demographic Yearbook 1965 (New York, 1966), Tables 14 and 17.

Table IX-4

ACTUAL AND HYPOTHETICAL AVERAGE AGE-SPECIFIC FERTILITY RATES FOR ELEVEN LATIN AMERICAN COUNTRIES COMBINED: 1960's[a]

(per thousand females)

	Age Groups						
	15-19	20-24	25-29	30-34	35-39	40-44	45-49
Actual Rates	124.11	311.14	320.68	256.53	195.10	76.25	19.07
Hypothetical Rates	12.89	136.78	159.93	122.57	81.44	33.33	3.45
Absolute Difference	111.22	174.36	160.75	133.96	113.66	42.92	16.25
Percent Difference[b]	89.6	56.0	50.1	52.2	58.3	56.3	82.5

[a]The actual and hypothetical age-specific fertility rates are the non-weighted averages of the rates for each of the eleven Latin American countries. (See Appendix IX, Table A-IX-1).

[b]The percent difference is the absolute difference divided by the actual rate and multiplied by 100.

19--90 percent--and a minimum reduction at age 25 to 29--50 percent. The differences increase with age after this last group.

Reduction of Birth Rates by Limiting Motherhood Ages

One way in which Latin America could have duplicated the European fertility pattern would have been by limiting the ages during which women could have children. One course would have been to set a maximum age for childbearing; an alternative would have been to set a minimum age. I will call the first course the United States model, and the second the Irish model. The names given the models reflect the characteristic age-specific fertility patterns in the two countries. The procedures for calculating the two limiting ages are given in Appendix IX.

The United States Model. To match the European pattern of fertility in relation to the level of life expectancy by this model, it was assumed that females would not have changed the spacing of their children, but simply that they would have stopped having them at a specified age. The maximum age at which females would have stopped bearing children in Latin American countries would have been very low, varying from 24 years in Venezuela to 29 years in Chile, and averaging 26 years for the eleven countries combined (Table IX-5, Column 2).[4]

The Irish Model. In this case also, it was assumed that females would not have altered the spacing of births while having children, but that they would have started bearing them at an age old enough to match the European fertility-mortality pattern. The minimum average age calculated for the eleven countries combined is 29, ranging between 27 in Chile and 32 in Costa Rica (see Table IX-5, Column 1).

Impossibility of Duplicating the European Pattern

The hypothetical means by which Latin America could have obtained the same relationship between life expectancy and birth rates as in Europe are seen to be unattainable when the required

---

[4] It should be remembered that the age limits calculated for each country depend on the expected hypothetical fertility level, which depends on the country's mortality level and on the actual age-specific fertility rates. Chilean age limits are most "reasonable," since the actual fertility rates are the lowest of the eleven countries considered. Costa Rica requires the highest minimum age because its hypothetical fertility level is very low (due to its low mortality) and its actual fertility rates very high.

Table IX-5

MINIMUM AND MAXIMUM AGES AT WHICH FEMALES WOULD HAVE BABIES IN ELEVEN LATIN AMERICAN COUNTRIES: 1960's[a]

	Minimum Age	Maximum Age
Country	(1)	(2)
Brazil	28.3	27.0
Chile	26.9	28.8
Costa Rica	32.4	25.2
El Salvador	28.9	25.1
Guatemala	28.1	25.7
Honduras	29.5	25.9
Mexico	29.7	26.4
Nicaragua	27.9	24.9
Panama	26.8	25.2
Paraguay	28.9	26.7
Venezuela	30.3	24.5
Average	28.9	25.9

[a]The minimum age is the age from which females could start having children in order to have the same birth rate as European countries, when the latter had the mortality level of Latin America in the 1960's, assuming actual Latin American age-specific fertility rates. The maximum age is the age after which females could not have babies, in order to duplicate the conditions described.

changes are analyzed in terms of the period of time during which such changes would have had to occur.

Birth Rates. An unprecedented decline in the birth rates of Latin American countries would have been necessary for these countries to reach the same mortality-fertility relationship as that registered in Europe. On the average, the crude birth rates in the 1960's would have had to be only 53 percent of actual levels. The Latin American crude birth rates (per thousand) would have had to decline at an annual average of .62 points during a 30-year period. No country in the world has manifested such a high annual average decline over such a long period of time.[5]

---

[5] The Soviet Union could possibly have had such a decline over a brief period. In 1910-14 Russia had a crude birth rate of approximately 43 per thousand. During the revolution, the birth rate was probably very low, but unfortunately there are no data for the revolutionary period. From 1924 to 1929 the birth rate was again over 40 per thousand, perhaps because of postponed births (Kuczynski, The Balance of Births and Deaths, Vol. II, pp. 134-135). The rate was 25.3 and 22.4 in 1955-59 and 1960-64, and averaged 19.7 per thousand in 1963-65 (United Nations, Demographic Yearbook 1966). Discounting the post-revolution baby boom, it required a little more than 40 years for the Soviet Union to reduce its birth rates to the level required in Latin America.

The birth rate in Taiwan in 1958 was 41.7 and in 1968 close to 29 per thousand. For ten years the decline was very rapid. But for the preceding 20 years the decline was not as fast as that required in Latin America. The island had a crude birth rate of 44.7 per thousand in 1935-39 (United Nations, Demographic Yearbook 1958), which decreased to 30.1 per thousand in 1966-68 (Taiwan Provincial Department of Health, Taiwan Population Studies Center, "Births Registered During January-May 1968" [Interim Report of Survey and Research Projects, No. 61], July 6, 1968), an annual average decline of .49 points. If the trend from 1956 to 1968 continues, however, or if the goal of the Fertility Control Program of a birth rate of 24.1 per thousand in 1971 is reached (L.P. Chow and T.D. Hsu, "The Progress of a Fertility Control Program in Taiwan," [Taiwan Provincial Department of Health, Taiwan Population Studies Center], October 1966), the Taiwanese birth rate decline would be the fastest in history. Unfortunately, from the crude birth rates in 1967 and 1968, it seems that the trend of the previous years is not continuing and that the goal of 24.1 will probably not be reached. The Fertility Control Program also has a goal of a total fertility rate of 2.937, but the ideal number of children in 1965 was 3.97 in a "province-wide Knowledge-Attitude-Practice (KAP)" (ibid.). Apparently Taiwanese females will have to reduce the "ideal" number of children, or

How many years passed before the crude birth rate in European countries fell from high levels--similar to those in Latin America--to low levels of 20 to 25 per thousand? At the beginning of this century, Western European countries already had crude birth rates of between 25 to 30 per thousand. Sweden's registers show that the crude birth rate was under 40 in 1721. Information for other European countries shows even lower rates than that a few years later. Finland surpassed Sweden in 1751-55, with a crude birth rate of 45.3 per thousand; by 1915-19, its crude birth rate had declined to 23.3 per thousand.[6] Poland's crude birth rate declined from 44.6 per thousand in 1895 to 27.1 in 1955-59 and 20.0 in 1960-64.[7]

The United States' crude birth rate declined from 44.3 to 21.3 per thousand in 70 years (1860-1930).[8] A Latin American country not included here--Argentina--reduced its crude birth rate from 42.9 per thousand in 1890-94 to 24.1 in 1955-59.[9] (During this period, Argentina received a large flow of immigrants from Europe, which was probably in part responsible for the changing attitude toward fertility.) In general, we can see that those countries which experienced a reduction of the crude birth rate of the magnitude hypothetically required for Latin American countries needed a much longer period of time than the 30-year period specified for Latin America.

Age-Specific Fertility Rates. Age-specific fertility rates in Latin America would have had to decline radically if the hypothetical crude birth rates were to be achieved. In general, it would have been necessary for this decline to exceed the decline of the crude birth rates, because of the age structure that

---

the goals of the program will not be reached by 1971. Probably even Taiwan, therefore, will not have as rapid a fertility decline as the one hypothetically required in Latin America.

[6] Kuczynski, The Balance of Births and Deaths, Vol. I, pp. 6-7, and Vol. II; Vielrose, Natural Movement of Population, Table 97, pp. 182-189; Kingsley Davis, "The World's Population Crisis," in R. Merton and R. Nisbet, eds., Contemporary Social Problems (2nd ed.; New York: Harcourt, Brace and World, Inc., 1966), pp. 347-408.

[7] Vielrose, Natural Movement of Population, and United Nations, Demographic Yearbook 1966.

[8] U.S. Department of Commerce, Bureau of the Census, Historical Statistics of the U.S., Colonial Times to 1957 (Washington, D.C., 1960), p. 23.

[9] Collver, Birth Rates, Table 5.

the hypothetical "B" populations would have had in the 1960's: a large proportion of females would have been in the peak reproductive ages.[10] The reduction of the age-specific rates (Table

---

[10]Because it was assumed in the projection that crude birth rates would have declined since the 1930's, the population over 30 would have remained the same. Furthermore, the percent in ages 20-29 in the hypothetical population would not have been much lower than in the actual population (16 percent in ages 20-24 and 9 percent in ages 25-29--Table VIII-4). As a consequence, not only would the proportion of potential mothers of reproductive ages have been large, but the age structure of the mothers would have been young as well. In other words, the proportion of young mothers whose fertility is highest--between age 20 and 30--would still have been very large, because the age structure would have been determined by high fertility conditions 30 years before. Such an age distribution of mothers tends to produce a higher birth rate than a population in which the proportion of mothers between the ages 20-30 is not so large. The percentages of females 20-29 in the total hypothetical "B" populations--both sexes --compared to the populations of selected European countries is as follows:

Latin American Hypothetical "B" Populations			Selected European Countries		
Brazil	(1960)	9.49	Denmark	(1962)	6.43
Chile	(1960)	9.70	Finland	(1963)	6.77
Costa Rica	(1963)	8.70	France	(1962)	6.08
El Salvador	(1967)	10.02	Iceland[a]	(1962)	6.36
Guatemala	(1964)	9.93	Ireland[a]	(1961)	6.35
Honduras	(1961)	9.23	Italy	(1962)	7.66
Mexico	(1960)	9.14	Malta[a]	(1963)	7.08
Nicaragua	(1963)	10.16	Netherlands[a]	(1963)	6.67
Panama	(1960)	8.95	Portugal[a]	(1960)	8.07
Paraguay	(1962)	9.64	Sweden	(1962)	6.05
Venezuela	(1961)	9.30	Yugoslavia[a]	(1961)	8.62

[a]Included in Table IX-3.

The average percentage for Latin America is 9.48; for countries in Table IX-3, 7.19; for the remaining European countries, 6.60 (data for Europe from United Nations, Demographic Yearbook 1962 and 1964). These percentages explain why the average hypothetical age-specific fertility rates for Latin American countries (Table IX-4) are lower than the average rates for European countries chosen as models (Table IX-3), although the average crude birth rates for both groups of countries were the same.

IX-4) would have necessitated a tremendous change of attitude toward reproduction in one generation. If Latin American countries had had very low fertility rates, it would have meant that most of the female population was using contraceptives. Is such a change during one generation possible? The degree of use of contraceptives required for such a decline will be determined by comparing Latin America with Taiwan and the United States. Taiwan has been chosen because of its recent family planning programs, and the United States because of the availability of data concerning contraceptive use.

We shall begin with Taiwan, more specifically with Taipei, where the family planning program has been concentrated. In Taipei, the government not only agrees with the family planning program, but also helps in its implementation, and the population in general, as well as the majority of religions practiced on the island,[11] accept the use of contraceptives. The family planning program is attempting to distribute intrauterine devices to all females who desire them, and most adult females appear to be accepting the devices. When the 1966 age-specific fertility rates of Taipei[12] were applied to the hypothetical "B" population for eleven Latin American countries combined (Tables VIII-4 and VIII-2), an average crude birth rate of 34 per thousand was obtained.

In the United States, the use of various contraceptives is common.[13] When the 1964 age-specific fertility rates for the

---

[11]Catholics form a very small group. The Taiwan Demographic Fact Book gives no information about religions, but an idea of the small proportion of Catholics can be obtained from the information about temples and shrines in three of the major cities (Taipei, Tainan, and Taichung). Of 234 temples and shrines in 1954, only nine were Catholic. (See U.S. Foreign Operation Administration, Mutual Security Mission to China, and National Taiwan University, Urban and Industrial Taiwan--Crowded and Resourceful [Taipei, September 1954], pp. 328-334.)

[12]The rates per thousand for each age group were: 42 for 15-19, 233 for 20-24, 256 for 25-29, 145 for 30-34, 57 for 35-39, 21 for 40-44, and 5 for 45-49 (from Taiwan, Department of Civil Affairs, 1966 Taiwan Demographic Fact Book, October 1967). The Latin American female population was that of Table VIII-4, Column (2). A comparison of the rates for Taipei with the hypothetical rates for Latin America in Table IX-4 shows the differences.

[13]The Population Council, "Roman Catholic Fertility and Family Planning: A Comparative Review of the Research Literature," Studies in Family Planning, No. 34 (October, 1968); Clyde V. Kiser, "The Indianapolis Study of Social and Psychological Factors

U.S. were applied to the Latin American populations, the results fluctuated between crude birth rates of 26.2 (Panama) and 28.7 (Nicaragua), with an average of 27.5 (Table IX-6). (In the United States, the crude birth rate for 1964 was 21.0.)[14]

The calculated crude birth rates of 34 and 27 per thousand from the two sets of age-specific fertility rates applied to Latin America were both higher than the hypothetical crude birth rate of 24 per thousand that Latin America needed to equal the crude birth rate of Europe at the same mortality level. In other words, to duplicate the European experience, Latin American age-specific fertility rates would have had to be even lower than those of the United States in 1964.

Obviously, a sharp decline of birth rates would have required as widespread a use of contraceptives as in the United States--or else abortion. Contraceptive methods would have been taught everywhere in each of the countries, and contraceptive devices would have been provided for the whole population. This would have necessitated a nationwide program supported by each government--a practical impossibility.[15]

Affecting Fertility" in C.V. Kiser, ed., Research in Family Planning (1962), pp. 149-166; Norman Ryder and Charles Westoff, "Use of Oral Contraception in the United States 1965," Science, 153, No. 3741 (Sept. 9, 1966): 1199-1205; R. Freedman, P. Whelpton, and A. Campbell, Family Planning, Sterility and Population Growth (New York: McGraw-Hill, 1959), Chaps. 3 and 6.

[14] U.S. Department of Health, Education and Welfare, Public Health Service, National Center for Health Statistics, Vital Statistics of the United States, 1966 (Washington, D.C., 1968), pp. 1-4.

[15] No Latin American country has a nationwide population policy. A few countries (i.e., Chile and Colombia) have started some family planning and/or birth control programs, but they have been applied only to small areas and only very recently. In general, the public does not accept such programs, and governments remain impassive or directly opposed to them. See, in Demography, Special Issue: Progress and Problems of Fertility Control Around the World, 5, No. 2 (1968), the following articles: Oscar Harkavy, Lyle Saunders, and Anna Southan, "An Overview of the Ford Foundation's Strategy for Population Work," pp. 550-551; Mario Jaramillo-Gomez, "Medellin: A Case of Strong Resistance to Birth Control," pp. 811-826; Walter Rodrigues, "Progress and Problems of Family Planning in Brazil," pp. 800-810; Mayone Stycos, "Opposition to Family Planning in Latin America: Conservative Nationalism," pp. 846-854. [continued]

Table IX-6

HYPOTHETICAL CRUDE BIRTH RATES FOR ELEVEN LATIN AMERICAN COUNTRIES ASSUMING SAME AGE-SPECIFIC FERTILITY RATES AS THE UNITED STATES IN 1964[a]

(per thousand)

Country	Hypothetical Crude Birth Rate
Brazil	27.5
Chile	27.6
Costa Rica	26.5
El Salvador	28.6
Guatemala	28.2
Honduras	27.2
Mexico	27.1
Nicaragua	28.7
Panama	26.2
Paraguay	27.5
Venezuela	27.4
Average[b]	27.5

[a]The U.S. age-specific fertility rates were .0347, .2199, .1794, .1039, .0500, .0138, and .0080 for each consecutive five-year age group from ages 15-49 (United Nations, Demographic Yearbook 1965, Table 17). The Latin American populations are from Chapter VIII, Appendix VIII, Table A-VIII-1, Column (2).

[b]Average is non-weighted.

Age at Marriage. Another possible way of reducing fertility without changing the age-specific fertility rates of married females would have been to set minimum ages for marriage, and to prevent intercourse outside of marriage. It is reasonable to assume that the minimum ages for marriage would be one year younger than the minimum ages at which females could start having children to obtain the same birth rate that European countries had at the same mortality level--that is, ages one year younger than those given in Table IX-5, Column (1). But to prevent marriage until these ages is a practical impossibility. For six Latin American countries with available information, the average proportion of single females in the 1960's at these hypothetical ages was only 32 percent of all women at these ages (see Table IX-7). It is not possible to force such a drastic change on a society in a generation. The other 68 percent of "ever married females" could not be expected to refrain from marital or sexual union up to the indicated age. Therefore, the non-contraceptive solution would also have been impossible.

Ideal or Desired Number of Children. The changes in fertility which would be necessary in order to give Latin America the same relationship between crude birth rates and life expectancy

---

Some articles in this issue of Demography can mislead the reader about birth control in Latin America. For instance, Deverell Colville, in "The International Planned Parenthood Federation--Its Role in Developing Countries," pp. 574-577, asserts, referring to Latin America (the whole area): "The prevalence of wide scale induced illegal abortion is so evident that there can be no question of any lack of motivation to curb fertility, and there is a general sentiment that contraception is preferable to abortion as a method of control...." (p. 577). Unfortunately, the author does not mention the sources showing "wide scale induced illegal abortion." The only available information about abortion in Latin America pertains to some of the larger cities. This information has been analyzed in an article by Requena (see--in the same issue of Demography--Mario Requena, "The Problem of Induced Abortion in Latin America," pp. 785-799). The article begins with the statement "In the majority of Latin American countries, induced abortion still constitutes the most widely used method or practice to avoid live birth...." Here Requena is making an assertion about the whole of Latin America, even though his data is limited to Mexico City, Bogota, Caracas, San Jose (Costa Rica), Buenos Aires, Panama City, and Rio de Janeiro.

A lack of governmental interest can be seen in the few countries that have made comments about population policies. These comments frequently reveal ambiguity about the goals of population control programs (see The Population Council, "Declaration of Population," Studies in Family Planning, No. 16 [January 1967]).

Table IX-7

PERCENTAGE OF FEMALES WHO WERE SINGLE AT THE HYPOTHETICAL MINIMUM AGES OF MARRIAGE IN SELECTED LATIN AMERICAN COUNTRIES: 1960's

Country	Census Year	Hypothetical Minimum Age at Marriage[a]	Percentage of Single Females at Hypothetical Minimum Age
Chile	1960	25.9	52.7
Costa Rica	1963	31.4	23.1
Honduras	1961	28.5	29.0
Mexico	1960	28.7	22.2
Panama	1960	25.8	39.5
Venezuela	1961	29.3	28.0
Average[b]		28.3	32.4

[a]These ages are one year less than those of Table IX-5, Column (1).

[b]The average is non-weighted.

that Europe manifested in the past would require a change in the number of children desired by Latin American females. A decline in the number of desired children presumes a vigorous population policy which would attempt to change the attitudes of the population toward fertility.[16] Such a program would probably be unsuccessful, given the difficulty of persuading people to reduce the number of children desired. For purposes of comparison, let us refer again to the United States. The number of children that an average family in the United States planned to have in the 1960's ("ideal," "intended," and/or "desired") is approximately

[16]Kingsley Davis, "Population Policy: Will Current Programs Succeed?" Science, 154, No. 10 (1967): 780-789.

If people themselves desire to have few children, they are able to find the means. England, Japan, France, Hungary, and Ireland, among other countries, reduced fertility without national programs to teach the use of contraceptives.

3.3.[17] The number of children considered ideal by the female population in certain Latin American cities varies considerably from one city to another, but the average for the largest cities in six of the countries was over 3.5 in 1964.[18] In the metropolitan area of Lima-Callao, the "preferred" number of children was over 4.1;[19] in Guatemala City, over 4.0.[20] These figures of ideal and preferred number of children come from the most urbanized areas of each country, and are almost certainly much lower than the average for the whole population. (Information on the ideal number of children for whole countries or rural areas is not available, except for data from a highland town in Peru, Huaylas, where the preferred number of children was 5.1.[21])

With such a high ideal number of children in Latin America, the population policy that would have been necessary to duplicate the European model would have required a reduction in the number of children desired of one or more child per family.[22]

---

[17]The number of children for the three different categories range between 3.2 and 3.4. See Judith Blake, "Family Size in the 1960's--A Baffling Fad?" Eugenics Quarterly, XIV, No. 1 (March 1967): 60-74, and N. Norman Ryder and Charles Westoff, "Relationship among Intended, Expected, Desired and Ideal Family Size: United States, 1965," Population Research (Center for Population Research, National Institute of Child Health and Human Development, National Institute of Health, March 1969), Table 4.

[18]Carmen A. Miro, "Some Misconceptions Disproved: A Program of Comparative Fertility Survey in Latin America" in B. Berelson, et al., eds., Family Planning and Population Programs (Chicago: University of Chicago Press, 1965), pp. 616-634. The cities and the respective ideal number of children are: Bogota, 3.64; Caracas, 3.50; Mexico, 4.20; Panama, 3.45; Rio de Janeiro, 2.22; San Jose (Costa Rica), 3.63. For this last city, Miguel Gomez, in Informe de la Encuesta de Fecundidad en el Area Metropolitana (San Jose, Costa Rica: Universidad de Costa Rica, Instituto Centroamericana de Estadistica, 1968), p. 58, Table 48, gives the ideal number of children as 4.1.

[19]Stycos, Human Fertility in Latin America, p. 149, Table 18.

[20]Michael Micklin, "Social and Economic Correlates of Ideal Family Size in Guatemala City." [Working Paper]

[21]Stycos, Human Fertility in Latin America, p. 149, Table 18.

[22]Using the previous figures for Latin American countries and the United States' "ideals," age-specific fertility rates, and crude birth rate, the reduction of one or more children was

Unfortunately, the ideal number of children seems to change slowly--at least it has in the United States since 1936.[23] Therefore, presumably it would have been difficult to obtain a reduction of one child per family in the desired number of children in Latin American countries during one generation. This change might be possible for certain minority groups of urban populations, but not for the whole country. Minority groups might have reached the educational level and acquired the social and economic aspirations to understand and appreciate the need for a reduced family. These conditions are lacking, and their attainment not readily foreseeable, in Latin American populations as a whole.

Conclusions

Various ways to obtain the decline of fertility necessary to have given Latin American countries the same crude birth rate as Europe at the same mortality level have been analyzed with the conclusion that the European pattern would not have been possible in Latin America. Among the several causes of this impossibility, one of the most important is the necessity of reducing fertility rapidly as a consequence of the rapid mortality decline. It is easier to influence a society in life-saving methods than to convince them of the long range need to prevent the inception of life. The reduction of mortality does not depend greatly on changes in those persons to be saved from death--they always wish to be saved. It depends principally on national public health programs, and on the medical knowledge of the most advanced nations of the world (see Chapter IV). The instinctive desire of any person is to continue to live; thus the application of sanitary and medical methods for reducing mortality is quickly accepted by any population.

Fertility reduction is just the opposite: it requires individual and subjective changes. Fertility in Latin America did not fall as mortality did because there were no national programs to send officers from house to house giving injections to produce temporary or permanent sterility, as there were programs to send officers from house to house spreading DDT or giving injections to children to prevent disease. There were no national programs designed to motivate the population to reduce family size, none to teach birth control or provide sex education; but there

---

estimated by assuming a direct, linear relationship between age-specific fertility rates, birth rates, and desired number of children. Such a linear relationship is not necessarily true, but it gives a fairly close estimate of the reduction needed.

[23] Blake, "Family Size in the 1960's," Table 3.

were many programs to teach disease prevention. No hospitals provided a woman with a safe abortion if she did not want a child, but many hospitals went to any length to save a life.

The lack of response of fertility to the mortality decline in Latin America has been the expected response, because of current cultural, educational, and economic characteristics of Latin American countries, together with the unusually rapid mortality decline. Under actual Latin American social and demographic conditions, the European mortality-fertility experience could not have been duplicated--the different period of time involved is a principal cause.

Appendix IX

Estimated Ages at Which Women Should Start--or Stop--Having Children in Order to Approach the Hypothetical Crude Birth Rates

The estimated age at which females could start having children in order to obtain the hypothetical crude birth rates of Table IX-1, Column (2), assumes that the age-specific fertility rates beyond that age would be the same as the actual rates in the 1960's. Before that age, no births would occur.

For this estimation, the hypothetical populations (Chapter VIII, Appendix VIII, Table A-VIII-1) will be used, since it is assumed that the reduction of fertility by changing the age at which females can start to be mothers will be a success.

The symbols used are: TB_x, the total number of births that would occur from age x of the mothers to the end of the fertile ages; N, the total hypothetical population (both sexes); $FN_{x,x+4}$, the female population in ages x to x+4; b, the hypothetical birth rate (Table IX-1, Column (2)); B, the total hypothetical births in the hypothetical population (B = b.N); and $\emptyset_{x,x+4}$, the actual age-specific fertility rates for age x, x+4 (Chapter VII, Table VII-4).

The required condition is that from age j, $TB_j = B$. For this purpose, the following summations can be obtained:

$$TB_s = \sum_{\substack{x=s \\ \Delta=5}}^{45} N_{x,x+4} \cdot \emptyset_{x,x+4} \qquad \text{(A-IX-1)}$$

$$TB_r = \sum_{\substack{x=r \\ \Delta=5}}^{45} N_{x,x+4} \cdot \emptyset_{x,x+4} \qquad \text{(A-IX-2)}$$

in such a way that

$$TB_s < B \leqq TB_r \qquad \text{(A-IX-3)}$$

As a consequence,

$$s > j \geqq r \quad \text{(A-IX-4)}$$

and by linear interpolation

$$j = r + \frac{B - TB_r}{TB_s - TB_r}(s-r) \quad \text{(A-IX-5)}$$

with j the age at which women could start having children.

The estimated age at which females should stop having children in order to obtain the hypothetical crude birth rate of Table IX-1, Column (2), assumes that the age-specific fertility rates up to that age would be the same as the actual rates in the 1960's. After that age, no births would occur. The procedure is exactly the same as before, but instead of accumulating births from age s or r to the end of the fertile age, the accumulation is now from the beginning of the fertile ages to age u or v. The desired age k will fall between v and u--$v \leqq k < u$.

Signifying the new cumulative number of births by AB_k,

$$AB_k = B = b.N \quad \text{(A-IX-6)}$$

then,

$$AB_u = \sum_{\substack{x=15 \\ \Delta=5}}^{u} N_{x,x+4} \cdot \emptyset_{x,x+4} \quad \text{(A-IX-7)}$$

and

$$AB_v = \sum_{\substack{x=15 \\ \Delta=5}}^{v} N_{x,x+4} \cdot \emptyset_{x,x+4} \quad \text{(A-IX-8)}$$

Similarly as before,

$$AB_u \leqq B < AB_v \quad \text{(A-IX-9)}$$

Therefore,

$$v \leqq k < u \quad \text{(A-IX-10)}$$

and

$$k = v + \frac{B - AB_u}{AB_v - AB_u}(u-v) \quad \text{(A-IX-11)}$$

Table A-IX-1

ACTUAL AND HYPOTHETICAL AGE-SPECIFIC FERTILITY RATES IN ELEVEN LATIN AMERICAN COUNTRIES: 1960's

(per thousand)

Rate	Age Groups						
	15-19	20-24	25-29	30-34	35-39	40-44	45-49
				BRAZIL			
Actual	96.55	282.17	300.87	242.97	198.19	85.02	18.90
Hypothetical	13.34	141.59	165.56	126.89	84.31	34.51	3.57
Absolute Difference	83.21	140.58	135.31	116.08	113.88	50.51	15.33
Percent Difference	86.18	49.82	44.97	47.78	57.46	59.41	81.11
				CHILE			
Actual	79.56	216.42	252.78	229.41	160.92	64.36	14.43
Hypothetical	13.09	138.87	162.37	124.45	82.69	33.84	3.50
Absolute Difference	66.47	77.55	90.41	104.96	78.23	30.52	10.93
Percent Difference	83.55	35.83	35.77	45.75	48.62	47.42	75.74
				COSTA RICA			
Actual	111.66	338.02	355.79	302.46	227.09	93.17	15.95
Hypothetical	11.10	117.74	137.67	105.51	70.11	28.69	2.97
Absolute Difference	100.56	220.28	218.12	196.95	156.98	64.48	12.98
Percent Difference	90.06	65.17	61.31	65.11	69.13	69.20	81.39

APPENDIX IX

EL SALVADOR

Actual	136.52	334.94	336.55	259.22	193.98	69.58	20.34
Hypothetical	12.64	134.17	156.88	120.24	79.89	32.70	3.38
Absolute Difference	123.88	200.77	179.67	138.98	114.09	36.88	16.96
Percent Difference	90.74	59.94	53.39	53.62	58.82	53.01	83.37

GUATEMALA

Actual	159.09	323.50	324.20	272.07	208.52	81.99	25.23
Hypothetical	14.43	153.11	179.03	137.21	91.17	37.31	3.86
Absolute Difference	144.66	170.39	145.17	134.86	117.35	44.68	21.37
Percent Difference	90.93	52.67	44.78	49.57	56.28	54.49	84.70

HONDURAS

Actual	147.29	320.45	347.53	287.64	216.33	89.54	23.91
Hypothetical	13.78	146.27	171.03	131.08	87.10	35.65	3.69
Absolute Difference	133.51	174.18	176.50	156.56	129.23	53.89	20.22
Percent Difference	90.64	54.35	50.79	54.43	59.74	60.19	84.58

MEXICO

Actual	102.41	299.32	319.15	257.75	210.21	90.32	19.91
Hypothetical	12.62	133.91	156.57	120.00	79.73	32.63	3.38
Absolute Difference	89.79	165.41	162.58	137.75	130.48	47.69	16.53
Percent Difference	87.68	55.26	50.94	53.44	62.07	63.87	83.04

NICARAGUA

Actual	145.42	368.67	376.74	248.06	191.16	65.67	20.42
Hypothetical	14.07	149.35	174.63	133.84	88.93	36.40	3.77
Absolute Difference	131.35	219.32	202.11	114.22	102.23	29.27	16.65
Percent Difference	90.32	59.49	53.65	46.05	53.48	44.58	81.56

Table A-IX-1 (continued)

Rate	Age Groups						
	15-19	20-24	25-29	30-34	35-39	40-44	45-49
PANAMA							
Actual	148.31	303.80	276.72	191.70	129.44	41.83	8.45
Hypothetical	12.18	129.27	151.15	115.85	76.97	31.50	3.26
Absolute Difference	136.13	174.53	125.57	75.85	52.47	10.33	5.19
Percent Difference	91.79	57.45	45.38	39.57	40.53	24.69	61.43
PARAGUAY							
Actual	104.33	297.78	293.08	265.93	216.26	92.62	22.68
Hypothetical	13.30	141.11	165.00	126.46	84.02	34.39	3.56
Absolute Difference	91.03	156.67	128.08	139.47	132.24	58.23	19.12
Percent Difference	87.25	52.61	43.70	52.45	61.15	62.87	84.31
VENEZUELA							
Actual	134.07	337.42	344.03	264.58	194.02	64.68	19.60
Hypothetical	11.23	119.16	139.33	106.79	70.95	29.04	3.00
Absolute Difference	122.84	218.26	204.70	157.79	123.07	35.64	16.60
Percent Difference	91.62	64.68	59.50	59.64	63.43	55.10	84.67

Source: See Table VII-4 for actual rates. For hypothetical rates see text.

PART V

CONCLUSION

Chapter X

SOME OF THE PRINCIPAL CONSEQUENCES OF THE RAPID MORTALITY DECLINE IN LATIN AMERICA

In Part II of this study we analyzed the unprecedented rapid mortality decline in Latin America from 1930 to 1960. The life expectancy at birth increased from 35 to 55 years in only one generation. By contrast, in Western Europe it took twice as long for life expectancies to increase from 40 to 55 years--a change 25 percent smaller than that in Latin America.

The high mortality of Latin American countries before the 1930's necessitated high fertility; otherwise they would not have survived. The situation up to the 1930's was essentially the same as in most other developing countries--high mortality, high fertility, and a moderate population growth rate of between 11 and 13 per thousand. Suddenly, in the 1960's--after a short period of only 30 years--the crude death rates of Latin American populations fell to levels of from 10 to 15 per thousand, causing the populations to grow at extremely high rates of over 30 per thousand. This vertiginous mortality decline is the primary cause of the present population imbalances.

The world population had always grown at a moderate rate--from the earliest recorded history to the seventeenth century. Since that time, however, the populations of some European countries have grown more rapidly, though the growth rates are still moderate. With industrialization and the concomitant development of medical science, mortality has fallen below previous levels. Viruses and bacteria are combatted with "laboratory" compounds, and the principal causes of death are no longer infectious-communicable diseases, but rather degenerative and chronic diseases.

In the industrialized countries, the process of mortality decline has taken place over a long period of time--long enough for the populations to adjust themselves to new conditions of life. The historical trends of crude birth and death rates show how the various countries have adjusted their demographic behavior from high to low mortality-fertility relationships. The European transition was a gradual process that took two or three centuries. The transition in Latin American countries, by contrast, began only recently, judging by the high mortality and fertility in the early 1900's. If these countries had been isolated from the rest of the world, the pace of their mortality decline and the resultant demographic transition would probably have been similar to that in Europe. But modern communications and the humanitarian policies of economically advanced benefactor nations and international organizations brought "external" or "imported" elements to Latin American populations which produced a rapid mortality decline.

No longer--as was the case in the 1930's--did 32 percent of the children die before their fifth birthday; no longer was there only a 50 percent chance of living to the age of 35. Latin American countries become so occupied with reducing mortality that to a large extent they forgot about fertility. Not until the censuses of the 1960's revealed that their populations were experiencing an unprecedented population increase did a general concern about the extremely high population growth rates in these countries develop among those involved in population studies. The same benefactor countries and international organizations that had helped to reduce mortality became aware of the tremendous imbalance being created in Latin America, and they began turning their attention to the reduction of fertility. But this awareness came too late; the imbalance already existed.

The public health programs which reduced mortality so drastically were not related to any long-range population policy; or if they were, the precautions taken were inadequate. The designers of the programs did not realize how easily mortality can be reduced in our modern age when it is at a very high level, and how difficult it is to reduce fertility in a short period of time--especially in Latin American countries where only a small proportion of the people have completed secondary school, and in which a high proportion of the people are bound to the doctrines of the Catholic Church concerning reproduction and artificial contraceptives. In addition, the designers of the programs did not take into account the difficulty of reducing the "desired" number of children in a population.[1] Under the prevailing social, economic,

---

[1] For example, in the United States the "ideal" number of children has remained practically constant since 1936 (see Blake, "Family Size in the 1960's," pp. 60-74).

The high number of children ever-born per mother given by Latin American censuses is related to the ideal number of children. In Chapter IX, it was concluded that the average ideal number of children in Latin America was over 4. Under the mortality conditions prevalent from 1925 to 1960 in the region, the author's calculations (using a deterministic model of family composition) indicate that in order to have 4.2 children alive at age 45-49 of the mother, the total number of children ever-born would have to be 6.1. The 1960 Mexican Census of Population gives an average number of children ever-born per mother aged 45-49 of 6.4. The same average number for Venezuela was 6.3 in 1950 and 6.0 in 1961.

and cultural conditions in Latin America, fertility could not appreciably decline, and it will be difficult to obtain a substantial reduction in the future. The consequences are already known: the actual populations in the 1960's were greater than any of the "high" forecasts based on information from the 1950's.[2] The conclusion to be drawn is not that mortality should have been left as it was, but rather that fertility should not have been left as it was. Along with public health programs to reduce mortality, there was an urgent need for education to teach the desirability of fewer children, and instruction in the use of birth control methods. In addition, provisions should have been made for national distribution of contraceptives.

Some of the consequences stemming from rapid mortality decline without a corresponding change in fertility were discussed in Part III. The pace of population growth generated by the demographic situation in Latin America in the 1960's was the greatest in world history. In addition, the age structure of the population became younger.

The acceleration of population growth as well as the change toward a younger population has tended to handicap economic and social development in Latin American societies. The change of the age structure has increased the number of people in non-active ages in relation to those in active ages. If labor participation rates of females had not risen, the number of dependents per worker would have increased. A decrease in fertility would have produced the opposite effect from that which mortality decline did--that is, a reduction in the number of dependents per worker.

The mortality decline has produced a school age population growing more rapidly than any other age group. Consequently, educational expenditures per worker in each country have tended to increase, even though only the same educational level has been maintained. Any improvement in education or any rise in student

---

From these numbers we can say that the completed fertility of the cohort aged 45-49 in the 1960's has been the desired fertility.

[2]Among the eleven Latin American countries considered in this study, the high forecasts for only four of them exceeded the actual populations in the 1960's. In these four cases, there was either over-estimation of the population in the 1950's or emigration during the decade. See Cesar Pelaez, "The Degree of Success Achieved in the Population Projections for Latin America Made Since 1950. Sources of Error. Data and Studies Needed in Order to Improve the Basis for Calculating Projections," World Population Conference 1965, 4 vols. (New York, 1967), 3: 27-33.

attendance will mean further increases. As Davis has pointed out, "The effort to combine health improvement with educational progress without controlling fertility is self-defeating."[3] A fertility decline would have helped significantly to better the education of Latin American populations.

If Latin American fertility had changed so as to maintain the European relationship between mortality and fertility, the situation in Latin America today would be completely different, and considerably more favorable to economic development. However, the required fertility change from the 1930's to the 1960's seems to have been impossible to attain. The Latin American mortality-fertility relationship is clearly different from that of Europe. It is unfortunate that the degree of difference is so considerable.

Social and economic progress with high fertility rates is almost impossible. If Latin American countries want to develop rapidly, the first measure to be taken--imposed by law if necessary--is the reduction of fertility. Incentives and motivations to reduce the number of births--actual, ideal, preferred, and/or desired--must be created. The sooner the fertility reduction comes about, the better it will be for the people in Latin America, both in terms of economic development and quality of life. Governments must remember that a nation's power is based not so much on the size of its population as on the quality of that population.

---

[3] Kingsley Davis, "The Population Impact on Children in the World's Agrarian Countries," Population Review, IX, Nos. 1 and 2 (January and July 1965): 28.

BIBLIOGRAPHY

Andre, Marius. El Fin del Imperio Español en América. Barcelona: Cultura Española, 1939.

Ariès, Philippe. Histoire des populations francaises et de leurs attitudes devant la vie depuis le XVIIIe siècle. Paris: Editions Self, 1948.

Arriaga, Eduardo. "Components of City Growth in Selected Latin American Countries," Milbank Memorial Fund Quarterly, XLVI, No. 2 (April 1968): 237-252.

_______. "The Effect of a Decline in Mortality on the Gross Reproduction Rate," Milbank Memorial Fund Quarterly, XLV, No. 3 (July 1967): 333-352.

_______. "New Abridged Life Tables for Peru: 1940, 1950-51 and 1961," Demography, III, No. 1 (July 1966): 218-237.

_______. New Life Tables for Latin American Populations in the Nineteenth and Twentieth Centuries. Berkeley: Institute of International Studies, University of California, 1968. [Population Monograph Series, No. 3]

_______. "Rural-Urban Mortality in Developing Countries: An Index for Detecting Rural Underregistration," Demography, IV, No. 1 (December 1967): 90-107.

_______, and Davis, Kingsley. "The Pattern of Mortality Change in Latin America," Demography, 6, No. 3 (August 1969): 223-242.

Barral Souto, J. and Somoza, J. "Construcción de una Tabla Abreviada de Mortalidad para la Argentina," Segundo Coloquio de Estadística. Córdoba, Argentina, 1953.

Becherelle, B., and Reyes, Jimenez. "Tablas de vida para México 1893 a 1956," Revista del Instituto de Salubridad y Enfermedades Tropicales, XVIII, No. 2 (June 1958): 81-136.

Beers, H.S. "Six-Term Formulas for Routine Actuarial Interpolation," Record of the American Institute of Actuaries, XXXIV (June 1945).

Bertillon, Jacques. La dépopulation de la France. Paris: Librairie Félix Alcan, 1911.

BIBLIOGRAPHY

Blake, Judith. "Family Size in the 1960's--A Baffling Fad?" Eugenics Quarterly, XIV, No. 1 (March 1967): 60-74.

Cabello, O., Vildosola, J., and Latorre, M. "Tablas de vida para Chile 1920, 1930 y 1940," Revista Chilena de Higiene y Medicina Preventiva, VIII, No. 3 (September 1946) and IX, No. 2 (June 1947).

Camisa, Zulma. "Assessment of Registration and Census Data on Fertility," Milbank Memorial Fund Quarterly, XLVI, No. 3 (July 1968), Part 2.

Case, Coghill C., Harley, J., and Pearson, J. The Chester Beatty Research Institute, Serial Abridged Life Tables, 1841-1960. London: The Chester Beatty Research Institute, Institute of Cancer Research, Royal Cancer Hospital, 1962.

Chile, Dirección de Estadística. Bulletin No. 12 (December 1962).

Chile, Dirección de Estadística y Censo. Demografía 1956. Santiago, Chile, 1956.

_______. Demografía 1960. Santiago, Chile, 1960.

_______. Demografía 1962. Santiago, Chile, 1962.

_______. Población del País, Características Básicas de la Población (Censo 1960). Santiago, Chile, 1964.

Chile, Servicio Nacional de Estadística y Censos. XII Censo General de Población y I de Vivienda, Tomo I Resumen del País. Santiago, Chile, 1956.

Chow, L.P., and Hsu, T.D. "The Progress of a Fertility Control Program in Taiwan." Taiwan Provincial Department of Health, Taiwan Population Studies Center, October 1966.

Coale, Ansley. "The Effects of Changes in Mortality and Fertility on Age Composition," Milbank Memorial Fund Quarterly, XXXIV, No. 1 (January 1956): 79-114.

_______, and Hoover, E. Population Growth and Economic Development in Low Income Countries. Princeton: Princeton University Press, 1958.

Collver, Andrew. Birth Rates in Latin America: New Estimate of Historical Trends and Fluctuations. Berkeley: Institute of International Studies, University of California, 1965. [Research Series No. 7]

_______. "Current Trends and Differentials in Fertility as

Revealed by Official Data," Milbank Memorial Fund Quarterly, XLVI (July 1968): 39-48.

Colville, Deverell. "The International Planned Parenthood Federation--Its Role in Developing Countries," Demography, Special Issue: Progress and Problems of Fertility Control Around the World, 5, No. 2 (1968): 574-577.

Davis, Kingsley. "The Amazing Decline of Mortality in Underdeveloped Areas," American Economic Review, 46 (1956): 305-318.

_______. "The Changing Demography of World Urbanization." Read at the Faculty Research Lecture, University of California, Berkeley, 1969.

_______. "Colonial Expansion and Urban Diffusion in the Americas," International Journal of Comparative Sociology, I, No. 1 (March 1960): 43-66.

_______. Human Society, 19th ed. New York: The Macmillan Co., 1965.

_______. "Population and Resources in the Americas," Proceedings of the Inter-American Conference on Conservation of Renewable Natural Resources. Denver, Colorado, September 7-20, 1948, pp. 88-96.

_______. "The Population Impact on Children in the World's Agrarian Countries," Population Review, IX, Nos. 1 and 2 (January and July 1956).

_______. "Population Policy: Will Current Programs Succeed?" Science, 154, No. 10 (1967): 780-789.

_______. "Population Trends and Policies in Latin America." In Some Economic Aspects of Post War Inter-American Relations. Austin: Institute of Latin American Studies, University of Texas, 1946.

_______. "The Sociology of Demographic Behavior." In Sociology Today, Problems and Prospects. Edited by R. Merton, L. Broom, and L. Cottrell. New York: Basic Books Inc., 1959.

_______. "The Theory of Change and Response in Modern Demographic History," Population Index, 29, No. 4 (October 1963): 345-366.

_______. "The Unpredicted Pattern of Population Change," Annals of the American Academy of Political and Social Science (May 1956): 53-59.

BIBLIOGRAPHY

_______. "The World Demographic Transition," Annals of the American Academy of Political and Social Science, 237 (January 1945): 1-11.

_______. "The World's Population Crisis." In Contemporary Social Problems. Edited by R. Merton and R. Nisbet, 2nd ed. New York: Harcourt, Brace and World, Inc., 1966.

_______. World Urbanization 1950-1970, Volume I: Basic Data for Cities, Countries and Regions. Berkeley: Institute of International Studies, University of California, 1969. [Population Monograph Series No. 4]

_______. World Urbanization 1950-1970, Volume II: Analysis of Trends, Relationships, and Development (forthcoming).

_______, and Blake, Judith. "Social Structure and Fertility: An Analytic Framework," Economic Development and Cultural Change, 4 (April 1956): 211-235.

Demeny, Paul. "Investment Allocation and Population Growth," Demography, 2 (1965): 203-232.

Durand, J.D. "World Population Estimates, 1750-2000," Proceedings of the World Population Conference, 1965, Vol. II. New York: United Nations, 1967.

Easterlin, Richard. "Effects of Population Growth on the Economic Development of Developing Countries," The Annals, 369 (January 1967): 98-108.

Feraud, L. "A propos du vieillissement d'une population," Proceedings of the World Population Conference, Vol. III. Rome: United Nations, 1954.

Frederiksen, Harald. "Determinants and Consequences of Mortality Trends in Ceylon," Public Health Reports, 76, No. 8 (August 1961).

_______. "Malaria Control and Population Pressure in Ceylon," Public Health Reports, 75, No. 10 (October 1960).

Freedman, R., Whelpton, P., and Campbell, A. Family Planning, Sterility and Population Growth. New York: McGraw-Hill, 1959.

Gini, Corrado. I Fattori Demografici, Dell'Evoluzione Delle Nazioni. New York: Italian Book Company, 1912.

Glass, David. "Malthus and the Limitation of Population Growth."

In Introduction to Malthus. Edited by D. Glass. New York: John Wiley and Sons, 1953.

Gomez, Miguel. Informe de la Encuesta de Fecundidad en el Area Metropolitana. San José, Costa Rica: Instituto Centro-americana de Estadística, Universidad de Costa Rica, 1968.

González Galé, José. Matemáticas Financieras (Segunda Parte) Elementos de Cálculo Actuarial. Buenos Aires: Librería El Ateneo Editorial, 1951.

Goodman, Leo. "On the Age-Sex Composition of the Population that Would Result from Given Fertility and Mortality Conditions," Demography, 4, No. 2 (1967): 423-442.

Gotz, Karl. Auswandern? Stuttgart: Friedrich Vorkwerk Verlag Stuttgart, 1951.

Guerra Iniguez, Daniel. La Revolución Americana. Caracas: Editorial Avila Gráfica S.A., 1949.

Gershenson, Harry. Measurement of Mortality. Society of Actuaries, 1961.

Hanke, Lewis, ed. The Origins of the Latin American Revolution 1808-1826. New York: Alfred A. Knopf, Inc., 1965.

Harkavy, O., Saunders, L., and Southan, A. "An Overview of the Ford Foundation's Strategy for Population Work," Demography, Special Issue: Progress and Problems of Fertility Control Around the World, 5, No. 2 (1968): 550-551.

Henderson, Robert. "Mathematical Theory of Graduation," Actuarial Studies, No. 4. New York: Actuarial Society of America, 1938.

________, and Sheppard, H.N. "Graduation of Mortality and Other Tables," Actuarial Studies, No. 4. New York: Actuarial Society of America, 1919.

Hubner, Gallo J. El Mito de la Explosión Demográfica. La Auto Regulación Natural de las Poblaciones. Buenos Aires: Joaquín Almendros Press, 1968.

Jaramillo-Gomez, Mario. "Medellin: A Case of Strong Resistance to Birth Control," Demography, Special Issue: Progress and Problems of Fertility Control Around the World, 5, No. 2 (1968): 811-826.

________, and Lodono, Juan B. "Rhythm, A Hazardous Contraceptive Method," Demography, 5, No. 1 (1968): 433-438.

BIBLIOGRAPHY

Johnson, Gwendolyn. "Health Conditions in Rural and Urban Areas of Developing Countries," Population Studies, XVII, No. 3 (March 1964): 293-309.

Keyfitz, Nathan. Introduction to the Mathematics of Population. Reading, Massachusetts: Addison-Wesley Publishing Co., 1968.

Kiser, Clyde V. "The Indianapolis Study of Social and Psychological Factors Affecting Fertility." In Research in Family Planning, edited by C. Kiser. Princeton: Princeton University Press, 1962.

Kuczynski, Robert. The Balance of Births and Deaths. Vol. I, The Macmillan Co., 1928; Vol. II, The Brookings Institution, Washington, D.C., 1931.

_______. The Measurement of Population Growth. London: Sidgwick and Jackson, Ltd., 1935.

Kuznets, Simon. "Population and Economic Growth," Proceedings of the American Philosophical Society, III, No. 3 (June 22, 1967): 170-193.

_______, Moore, W., and Spengler, J., eds. Economic Growth: Brazil, India, Japan. Durham, N.C.: Duke University Press, 1955.

Lorimer, F. "Dynamics of Age Structure in a Population with Initially High Fertility and Mortality," Population Bulletin No. 1 (December 1951). New York: United Nations, pp. 31-41.

Loyo, G. Población y Desarrollo Economica. Mexico: Tipografica Londres, 1963.

Micklin, Michael. "Social and Economic Correlates of Ideal Family Size in Guatemala City." Unpublished paper.

Miro, Carmen. "The Population of Latin America," Demography, I, No. 1 (1964): 15-41.

_______. "Some Misconceptions Disproved: A Program of Comparative Fertility Survey in Latin America." In Family Planning and Population Programs. Edited by B. Berelson et al. Chicago: The University of Chicago Press, 1965.

Mortara, Giorgio. "Estudos sobre a Utilizaçao das Estadisticas do Movimiento da Populaçao do Brazil," Revista Brasilera de Estadistica, Year II, No. 7 (July-September 1941): [illegible]3-538.

McKeown, Thomas, and Record, R.G. "Reasons for the Declining of

Mortality in England and Wales during the Nineteenth Century," Population Studies, 16 (November 1962): 94-122.

Pelaez, Cesar. "The Degree of Success Achieved in the Population Projections for Latin America Made Since 1950. Sources of Error. Data and Studies Needed in Order to Improve the Basis for Calculating Projections," Proceedings of the World Population Conference 1965, Vol. III. New York: United Nations, 1967.

Penrose, E.F. Population Theories and Their Application. Stanford: Food Research Institute, Stanford University, 1934.

The Population Council. "Declaration of Population," Studies in Family Planning, No. 16 (January 1967).

_______. "Roman Catholic Fertility and Family Planning: A Comparative Review of the Research Literature," Studies in Family Planning, No. 34 (October 1968).

Population Reference Bureau, Inc. World-wide War on Malaria. Washington, D.C.: Population Bulletin (March 1958).

Rele, J.R. Fertility Analysis through Extension of Stable Population Concepts. Berkeley: Institute of International Studies, University of California, 1967. [Population Monograph Series, No. 2]

Requena, Mario. "The Problem of Induced Abortion in Latin America," Demography, Special Issue: Progress and Problems of Fertility Control Around the World, 5, No. 2 (1968): 785-799.

_______. "Social and Economic Correlates of Induced Abortion in Santiago, Chile," Demography, 2 (1965): 33-49.

Retel-Laurentin, Anne. "Influence de certaines maladies sur la fécondité, un exemple africain," Population, 22, No. 5 (September-October 1967): 841-860.

Rodrigues, Walter. "Progress and Problems of Family Planning in Brazil," Demography, Special Issue: Progress and Problems of Fertility Control Around the World, 5, No. 2 (1968): 800-810.

Rosenblat, Angel. La Población Indígena y el Mestizaje en America. Buenos Aires: Editorial Nova, Biblioteca Americanista, 1954.

Russell, P.F. Man's Mastery of Malaria. Oxford University Press, 1955.

BIBLIOGRAPHY

Ryder, N. Norman, and Westoff, Charles. "Relationship among Intended, Expected, Desired and Ideal Family Size: United States, 1965," Population Research. Center for Population Research, National Institute of Child Health and Human Development, National Institute of Health (March 1969).

_______. "Use of Oral Contraception in the United States 1965," Science, 153, No. 3741 (September 9, 1966): 1199-1205.

Sauvy, Alfred. Richesse et population. Paris: Bibliothèque Economique, Seconde Edition Revue, 1944.

_______. Teoria General de la Población. Madrid: Editorial Aguilar, 1957.

_______. "Le vieillissement des populations et l'allongement de la vie," Population, No. 4 (1954): 675-682.

Somoza, Jorge. "Trends of Mortality and Expectation of Life in Latin America," Milbank Memorial Fund Quarterly, XLIII, No. 4 (October 1965): 219-233.

Statistiska Centralbyran. Historisk Statistik for Sverige (1720-1950). Stockholm, 1955.

_______. Statistisk Arsbok. (Several years.)

Stolnitz, George. "A Century of International Mortality Trends: I," Population Studies, IX, No. 9 (July 1955): 24-55.

_______. "Recent Mortality Trends in Latin America, Asia and Africa," Population Studies, XIX, No. 2 (November 1965): 117-138.

Stycos, Mayone. Human Fertility in Latin America. Ithaca, N.Y.: Cornell University Press, 1964.

_______. "Opposition to Family Planning in Latin America: Conservative Nationalism," Demography, Special Issue: Progress and Problems of Fertility Control Around the World, 5, No. 2 (1968): 846-854.

Taeuber, Irene B. The Population of Japan. Princeton, N.J.: Princeton University Press, 1958.

Taiwan, Department of Civil Affairs. 1966 Taiwan Demographic Fact Book. October 1967.

Taiwan, Foreign Operation Administration, Mutual Security Mission to China, and National Taiwan University. Urban and Industrial Taiwan--Crowded and Resourceful. Taipei, September 1954.

Taiwan, Taiwan Provincial Department of Health, Taiwan Population Studies Center. "Births Registered During January-May 1968," Interim Report of Survey and Research Projects, Report No. 61 (July 6, 1968).

Thompson, Warren S. Population Problems, 4th ed. New York: McGraw-Hill Book Co., 1953.

United Nations. The Aging of Populations and Its Economic and Social Implications. New York, 1956.

_______. "The Cause of the Aging of Populations: Declining Mortality or Declining Fertility?" Population Bulletin No. 4 (December 1954).

_______. Demographic Yearbook 1950. New York, 1951.

_______. Demographic Yearbook 1953. New York, 1954.

_______. Demographic Yearbook 1956. New York, 1957.

_______. Demographic Yearbook 1958. New York, 1959.

_______. Demographic Yearbook 1959. New York, 1960.

_______. Demographic Yearbook 1962. New York, 1963.

_______. Demographic Yearbook 1963. New York, 1964.

_______. Demographic Yearbook 1964. New York, 1965.

_______. Demographic Yearbook 1965. New York, 1966.

_______. Demographic Yearbook 1966. New York, 1967.

_______. Handbook of Vital Statistics Methods. Series F, No. 7. New York, 1955.

_______. Human Resources of Central America, Panama, and Mexico, 1950-1980. Prepared by Luis J. Ducoff. ST/TAD/K/LAT/1, E/CN.12/548. New York, 1960.

_______. Methods for Population Projections by Sex and Age. Manual III, ST/SOA/Series A, Population Studies No. 25. New York, 1956.

_______. Migration, Urbanization and Economic Development. Vol. IV of World Population Conference, 1965. New York, 1967.

_______. The Population of South America 1950-1980. ST/SDA/ Series A, Population Studies No. 21. New York, 1955.

_______. Sex and Age of International Migrants: Statistics for 1918-1947. New York, 1953.

U.S., Department of Commerce, Bureau of the Census. Historical Statistics of the U.S., Colonial Times to 1957. Washington, D.C.

U.S., Department of Health, Education, and Welfare, Public Health Service, National Center for Health Statistics. Vital Statistics of the United States, 1966. Washington, D.C., 1968.

Valaoras, V.G. "Patterns of Aging of Human Populations." In The Social and Biological Challenge of Our Aging Population. New York: Columbia University Press, 1950.

Vielrose, Egon. Elements of the National Movement of Population. Pergamon Press, 1965.

Whelpton, P.K., and Kiser, Clyde V., eds. Social and Psychological Factors Affecting Fertility. Vols. I-V. New York: Milbank Memorial Fund, 1958.

Willcox, Walter. "Increase in the Population of the Earth and of the Continents." In International Migrations, Vol. II. Washington, D.C.: National Bureau of Economic Research, 1931.

World Health Organization. Epidemiological Yearbook 1961.